The Medi-Cal ADVANTAGE

How To Save The Family Home From The Cost Of Nursing Home Care

F. Douglas Lofton & Mellanese S. Lofton

ISBN 0-9667737-0-5

Copyright ©1999 by Lailabela Press

Printed in the United States of America

Lailabela Press
2020 Columbus Pkwy. #4
Benicia, California 94510

ISBN 0-9667737-0-5

DEDICATION

This book is dedicated to the caregivers of the frail elderly who, on a daily basis, give of so much of themselves to care for others.

ACKNOWLEDGEMENTS

We, the authors, would like to especially thank Robin M. Lofton-Koponen for her tireless efforts in editing this book. Her assistance in this project, including the use of her keen eye, skillful pen, and insightful comments were invaluable to us in writing this book.

We also thank David Paulley of Ram Graphics in Oakland, CA, for the outstanding quality of his work in the book's design and production. His diligence and thoroughness is greatly appreciated.

Finally, we thank the California Department of Health Services and the Solano County Welfare Department for their assistance in providing critical information on the Medi-Cal regulations and their practical implementation at the county level.

About The Book

The book, The Medi-Cal Advantage, was designed using a Mac. The photograph of the 3 people in the Illustration sitting on the "3D desk" on the front cover of the book is of the artist, David Paulley, and his ever-loving parents, Don and Bonnie Paulley of Casper, Wyoming. Thank you Doug, for allowing me to "render" my parents for the benefit of all who will benefit from The Medi-Cal Advantage.

TABLE OF CONTENTS

Table of Contents

Table of Contents

Table of Contents

HOW TO USE THE MEDI-CAL ADVANTAGE

The Medi-Cal Advantage is both a REFERENCE TOOL and a WORKBOOK. As such, it provides you with the necessary planning tools to save your home and other assets from the cost of nursing home care.

I. USING THE MEDI-CAL ADVANTAGE AS A REFERENCE TOOL

The Medi-Cal Advantage is a reference tool in that it is written in a easy-to-follow question and answer format so that you, the reader, can quickly receive the information that you need without having to read the entire book. In order to find the answers to your Medi-Cal questions, merely locate the question in the Table of Contents, and then look up the corresponding page number for the question and answer in the book. For example, suppose your question is the following:

IF MY LOVED ONE NEEDS TO ENTER A NURSING HOME, WHAT IS THE MAXIMUM AMOUNT OF ASSETS SHE CAN OWN AND QUALIFY FOR MEDI-CAL BENEFITS?

STEP #1: Turn to the TABLE OF CONTENTS in order to find the appropriate *Chapter* and *Section*. For this question, you would find CHAPTER TWO: THE MEDI-CAL ELIGIBILITY RULES. You will also find that each chapter is divided into two sections: Single Persons and Married Persons. If you are single, you only need to refer to the section for single persons. If you are married, you only need to refer to the section for married persons.

STEP #2: After you have found the appropriate chapter and section in the Table of Contents, then identify your specific question and the corresponding page number in the book where the question is located and answered. For single persons, the question regarding the eligibility requirements is located and answered on page 21.

Do not worry that your question may not be located in the book. You are very likely to find your question, since the questions listed and answered are based on the questions we have received from many clients over a period of years.

II. USING THE MEDI-CAL ADVANTAGE AS A WORKBOOK:

The Medi-Cal Advantage is also a workbook in that it provides both married persons and single persons with two essential forms to complete: 1) The Medi-Cal Eligibility Determination Worksheet, and 2) The Asset Protection Strategies Checklist. Collectively, these completed forms will reveal your current Medi-Cal eligibility status and, if you are ineligible, they will greatly assist you in planning to become eligible while minimizing the spend down of your assets.

(1) THE MEDI-CAL ELIGIBILITY DETERMINATION WORKSHEET.

The Medi-Cal Advantage provides you with the ability to determine if you are currently eligible for Medi-Cal. In order to determine your Medi-Cal eligibility status, you can use **The Medi-Cal Eligibility Determination Worksheet** located in the book's appendix (see Fig. 1). The Worksheet has three columns: 1.) The Type of Asset; 2.) The Category of the Asset—Exempt or Non-Exempt; and 3.) The Value of the Asset. The first two columns regarding the Type and Category of the asset are completed for you. You merely need to state the value of your assets in the blank third column. Once completed, the Worksheet will reveal whether you are currently eligible or ineligible for Medi-Cal. If you are ineligible, the Worksheet will identify the reason why you are ineligible for Medi-Cal. For example, the Worksheet might reveal that the you are ineligible for Medi-Cal because you have too much cash.

(2) THE ASSET PROTECTION STRATEGIES CHECKLIST

If you are currently ineligible for Medi-Cal, refer to **The Asset Protection Strategies Checklist**, also located in the book's Appendix (see Fig. 2). This form consists of a checklist of strategies that you can implement in order to become eligible for Medi-Cal, while minimizing the spend down of your assets. Each strategy listed is designed to address a particular Medi-Cal eligibility problem. Further, each strategy has a corresponding page number in the book where the use of strategy is discussed in detail.

For example, suppose The Medi-Cal Eligibility Determination Worksheet reveals that you are ineligible because you have too much cash; you can do the following:

STEP #1: Refer to the Asset Protection Strategies Checklist in the Appendix and look under the section: "Strategies to Protect Cash." For single persons, there are four strategies listed. For married persons, five strategies are listed.

STEP #2: Turn to the corresponding page number(s) in the book where each of these strategies are discussed in detail. After reading the discussion, select the most appropriate strategy for your situation. Be sure to check each strategy that you select in the corresponding box in the checklist so that you have a record of exactly what strategies you plan to implement.

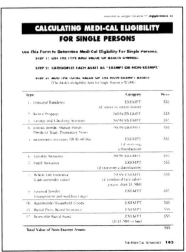

Fig. 1
Calculating Medi-Cal
Eligibility for single persons.

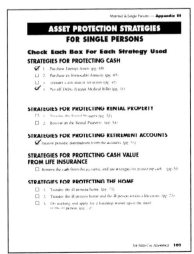

Fig. 2
Asset Protection Strategies
for single persons.

Publisher's Note

This publication is designed to provide accurate information with regard to the subject matter covered. It is sold with the understanding that the publisher is not engaged in rendering legal, financial, tax, or other professional advice to the reader. If the advice of a professional is necessary, a competent professional should be sought to provide such services.

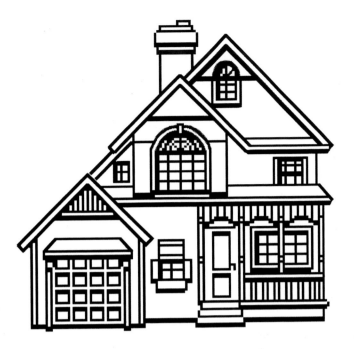

The Medi-Cal ADVANTAGE

How To Save The Family Home From The Cost Of Nursing Home Care

INTRODUCTION

Albert and Martha are seventy-five years old. They have been married for more than fifty years. Albert retired from his company after nearly forty years of service. Martha worked part-time and was a dedicated homemaker. They own their home, free and clear, and have approximately $100,000 in savings. Between their savings accounts, social security and retirement pensions, they had enough income and assets to enjoy a comfortable retirement.

Then Albert had to be placed in a nursing home. Albert had Alzheimer's disease. When Martha could no longer take care of Albert, she reluctantly placed him in a nursing home. To her surprise, she discovered that neither Medicare nor their private health insurance plan covered his nursing home expenses.

Today, Martha pays Albert's annual nursing home bill of $40,000 from their life savings. At this rate, Albert and Martha will exhaust their $100,000 in savings within a few years. The thought of divorcing Albert, after fifty happy years of marriage, to financially protect herself is unthinkable to Martha. Consequently, in a few years, Martha may have to sell their home to pay for her husband's care. With the potential loss of their home and savings, Martha and Albert face a future in poverty.

Albert and Martha are not alone. This hypothetical story describes an emotional and financial crisis that an increasing number of seniors and their families are confronting daily.

AGING AND INCAPACITY: A GROWING PHENOMENON

People are living longer. In fact, the elderly population is the fastest growing segment of the U.S. population today. Between 1980 and 1990, the percentage of persons aged eighty-five and older increased by nearly 50 percent. This trend is expected to accelerate as the baby boom population ages. According to the U.S. Administration on Aging, the number of Americans aged sixty-five and older will more than double by the year 2030.

As the U.S. population grows older, there has been a corresponding increase in the number of Americans who need long-term nursing home care. According to the U.S. Accounting Office, more than seven million Americans aged sixty-five and over are receiving some form of long-term care due to a chronic condition, trauma or illness that limits their ability to carry out personal care tasks such as feeding, bathing, or dressing.

Today, over 25 percent of all Americans aged sixty-five and over are expected to spend sometime in a nursing home. According to the U.S. Administration on Aging, the number of Americans needing long-term care is expected to double in size to fourteen million persons in the next twenty-five years.

Unfortunately, the cost of long-term care, particularly nursing home care, has placed an enormous financial hardship upon many senior citizens and their families. In California, nursing home care cost exceeds $40,000 per year. Such enormous health care costs have caused many seniors to lose their homes and forced many seniors to deplete their life savings. Once impoverished, most seniors must rely on Medi-Cal benefits to cover the cost of their nursing home care.

THE NEED FOR MEDI-CAL PLANNING

Medi-Cal is a joint federal and state health care assistance program that pays the cost of the long-term care needed by most nursing home patients. In fact, half of all nursing home patients in California rely on Medi-Cal benefits to pay for the cost of their care. Unfortunately, many seniors trying to get Medi-Cal benefits will encounter many legal and financial hurdles. Unlike Medicare, Medi-Cal has strict legal and financial requirements for eligibility. For many seniors, these eligibility requirements are seemingly insurmountable—short of becoming impoverished.

Based on our experience in advising clients about Medi-Cal, obtaining Medi-Cal benefits without the ill person or their spouse becoming impoverished is possible. However, obtaining Medi-Cal benefits without becoming impoverished requires Medi-Cal planning.

Medi-Cal Planning involves purchasing, transferring or liquidating assets to qualify for Medi-Cal benefits to pay for the cost of nursing home care. Effective Medi-Cal Planning can allow seniors to preserve a substantial portion of their estate while enabling their loved ones to qualify for Medi-Cal benefits. Indeed, Medi-Cal planning is becoming as essential to the preservation of one's estate as are the traditional areas of tax and estate planning.

USING "THE MEDI-CAL ADVANTAGE"

We wrote the "Medi-Cal Advantage" to enable caregivers of the elderly to become "Medi-Cal Planners" for their loved ones. We wrote it especially for caregivers because they are usually placed in the difficult position of taking care of the legal and health care needs of their loved ones—and often simultaneously. Caregivers typically include friends and family members who assist their incapacitated loved one on a variety of tasks, such as providing personal care, bookkeeping, shopping, and transportation. However, caregivers also include professionals who provide services to the frail elderly in a variety of contexts. Professional caregivers include social workers, conservators, ombudsmen, doctors, nurses, financial planners, attorneys, and accountants.

The purpose of "The Medi-Cal Advantage" is to give caregivers the critical information they will need to protect their loved one's assets from catastrophic nursing home costs. Each Chapter of the book is divided into two sections:

> I   Medi-Cal for Married Persons, and
>
> II   Medi-Cal for Single Persons.

The division of this book is necessary since the rules regarding married and single Medi-Cal recipients often differ.

The information is organized in a question-and-answer format and in "non-legalese" so that the reader can obtain answers to their questions quickly and clearly. The questions addressed in this book are based on the most common questions presented by caregivers during our years advising clients on Medi-Cal problems.

This book contains a number of tools that caregivers should find useful. These tools include practical forms, such as a Medi-Cal Eligibility Determination Worksheet, and sample Medi-Cal Plans. We have also included True/False review questions, along with detailed explanation of the answers, in order to reinforce the rules and concepts learned in the chapters.

Although designed to be an information resource for caregivers, it is not intended to be a substitute for legal and/or financial advice. "The Medi-Cal Advantage" is not, and cannot be, a guide to all the rules and regulations concerning Medi-Cal for nursing home care. Because the Medi-Cal laws and regulations are extremely complex, dynamic, and occasionally contradictory, implementing a Medi-Cal Plan without first obtaining professional advice can result in unintended legal and financial consequences. Therefore, **caregivers who develop a Medi-Cal Plan for their loved ones should consult an Elder Law or Estate Planning Attorney before implementing the Plan.** In consulting an attorney, it is highly recommended that the attorney review the Plan. Also, we recommend that a tax lawyer or Certified Public Accountant (CPA) be consulted regarding any tax consequences which could result from Medi-Cal Planning.

The central message of "The Medi-Cal Advantage" is this: **Your loved one's need not, and should not become impoverished because of catastrophic illness.** In our years working as elder law attorneys, we have helped many couples like Albert and Martha, as well as single individuals. We hope and trust that this book will also help your loved ones protect the family home and other assets that they have worked so hard over the years to obtain.

—F. Douglas Lofton, Esq.
—Mellanese S. Lofton, Esq.

CHAPTER 1

FINANCING THE COST OF NURSING HOME CARE

This Chapter Covers:

Methods of Financing Nursing Home Care

Types of Nursing Home Care

Medicare vs. Medi-Cal

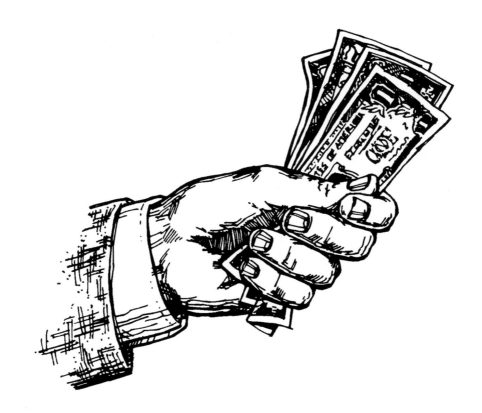

INTRODUCTION

This introductory chapter explores the various options of financing nursing home care. It begins with a discussion of the shortcomings of traditional health insurance and long-term care insurance. However, the chapter focuses on the two principal government programs that finance the cost nursing home care: Medicare and Medi-Cal. This chapter highlights the significant differences between these programs, including the different eligibility requirements, and explains why most long-term nursing patients rely on Medi-Cal benefits as opposed to Medicare to pay for the cost of their care.

IF MY LOVED ONE ENTERS A NURSING HOME, WILL TRADITIONAL HEALTH INSURANCE FINANCE THE COST OF CARE?

No. In California, nursing home care costs approximately $3,500 per month, or $42,000 per year.

Unfortunately, traditional health insurance plans do not provide coverage for long-term care in a nursing home. This is a tragic discovery for many caregiver relatives who are handling the financial affairs of their loved ones.

IF TRADITIONAL HEALTH INSURANCE DOES NOT FINANCE THE COST OF NURSING HOME CARE, WHO WILL PAY THE COST?

There are several methods of financing the cost of nursing home care. One obvious method is to pay the nursing home from one's own financial resources, which include one's savings and income. However, few elderly Californians can afford to pay this cost over an extended period without completely depleting all of their funds. In fact, many elderly Californians have lost their homes and depleted their savings as a consequence of financing the cost of their nursing home care.

Another method is to have long-term care insurance finance the cost of care. The use of long-term care insurance is growing as more people become familiar with the existence of these types of policies. Unfortunately, the monthly premiums are cost-prohibitive for most elderly persons, many of whom are living on a fixed income. Moreover, the persons who are already in a nursing home, or will most likely need nursing home care in the immediate future, will not usually qualify. Finally, there are two public assistance programs that will finance the cost of nursing home care. These programs are Medicare and Medi-Cal.

WHAT IS MEDICARE?

Medicare is a federal health insurance program for the elderly and disabled. If one is eligible to receive Social Security, one is eligible to receive Medicare. There are no financial eligibility requirements to receive Medicare except for a small monthly premium that is required to receive certain outpatient services.

Unfortunately, Medicare only pays for the type of care that is needed by a small minority of long-term nursing home patients. Under the laws regulating the program, Medicare will only pay for the cost of nursing home care for patients who need "skilled care". Skilled care is a level of care that requires the expertise of a doctor, nurse, or therapist. Examples of skilled care include physical therapy or rehabilitative therapy. Nursing home patients who are in a facility for longer than three months typically do not need skilled care; rather, they need "custodial care".

Custodial care is health care that involves ordinary daily activities such as feeding, bathing, and dressing. Custodial care is particularly needed by patients who suffer from dementia such as Alzheimer's disease. For example, an Alzheimer's patient can be physically healthy, and therefore would not need skilled care such as physical and rehabilitative therapy. However, the degenerative brain condition caused by the disease renders him or her unable to care for himself or herself. **Medicare only pays for nursing home care for a limited time. This is because Medicare only covers the costs nursing home care while the patient needs skilled care.** Therefore, Medicare, as a practical matter, covers only a small portion of most long term patients' nursing home costs.

Not only is Medicare assistance limited to nursing home patients who need skilled care, the program will finance the cost of this care for only a limited period of time. Medicare will only pay the daily cost of care from the third through the twenty-first day in which the patient resides in the nursing home and needs skilled care. From the twenty-second day to the hundredth day, the patient (or patient's family) must pay approximately $90.00 per day. Medicare will pay the additional costs. The daily payment for which the patient is responsible for is known as his or her "co-payment." However, Medicare supplemental insurance will finance this co-payment. After the hundredth day of skilled care per calendar year and illness, the patient (or patient's family) is responsible for the entire cost of nursing home care.

WHAT IS MEDI-CAL?

Medi-Cal is the federal Medicaid program implemented in California. Medi-Cal will finance the cost of nursing home care as long as the patient meets certain financial eligibility requirements. Under the Medi-Cal regulations, the patient must attempt admission to (or already reside in) a Skilled Nursing Facility (SNF) or an Intermediate Care Facility (ICF), and the facility itself must be Medi-Cal certified.

Unlike the Medicare program, the Medi-Cal program will finance the cost of custodial nursing home care for patients who qualify financially. As a consequence, Medi-Cal is the most common method of financing nursing home care. In fact, Medi-Cal finances the cost of care for half of all nursing home patients in California.

†The Medi-Cal
eligibility requirements
between married and
single persons differ
substantially because
the current rules are
designed to protect a
well spouse from
impoverishment. Since
there is no spouse to
protect in the case of a
single person, the
financial eligibility
requirements are much
more stringent.

WHO QUALIFIES FOR MEDI-CAL BENEFITS?

Adults who are "medically indigent" and reside in either a Skilled Nursing Facility (SNF) or an Intermediate Care Nursing Facility (ICF) qualify for Medi-Cal benefits. The determination of "medically indigent" depends upon whether the person is married or single. **If the ill person is married, he or she may qualify for Medi-Cal benefits if the value of the married couple's assets does not exceed $83,960 in 1999.** This asset limitation is adjusted each year for the cost of living. **A single person is "medically indigent" if the value of his or her assets does not exceed $2,000.**†

DO ALL NURSING HOMES ACCEPT MEDI-CAL?

No. All nursing homes do not accept Medi-Cal. However, facilities that do accept Medi-Cal will be "Medi-Cal Certified" by the State. A nursing home that is Medi-Cal Certified means that it is authorized to have Medi-Cal patients. If your loved one is in a facility that is not certified to have Medi-Cal patients, he or she cannot eventually convert to Medi-Cal. Thus, in choosing a nursing home for the ill spouse, it is important to inquire as to whether the facility is Medi-Cal Certified. The admissions officer of the facility can provide this information.

CHAPTER 1: SUMMARY

- Traditional health insurance plans do not provide coverage for long-term care in a nursing home.

- Medicare is a federal health insurance program for the elderly and disabled. Although Medicare does cover nursing home costs, it only does so when the ill person needs "skilled care." Examples of skilled care include physical therapy and rehabilitative therapy. Skilled care is only needed by a small minority of nursing home patients.

- Medi-Cal is a federal and state health insurance program. Unlike Medicare, the Medi-Cal program covers nursing home care costs when the ill person needs "custodial care." Examples of custodial care include feeding, bathing, and dressing. Custodial care is the type of care needed by most nursing home patients, particularly those who suffer from dementia.

- Medi-Cal is a program for the "medically indigent." Consequently, the ill person must meet the financial eligibility requirements of the program in order to qualify for the Medi-Cal benefits. If the ill person is married, the ill spouse could qualify for Medi-Cal benefits if the value of the married couple's assets does not exceed $83,960. A single person could qualify for Medi-Cal benefits if the value of his or her assets does not exceed $2,000.

- In order for Medi-Cal to finance the nursing home costs of your loved one, he or she must reside in a nursing home that is "Medi-Cal Certified."

CHAPTER 2

MEDI-CAL ELIGIBILITY RULES

This chapter covers the following:

Medi-Cal Financial Eligibility Limits

Exempt vs. Non-Exempt Assets

Method of Calculating Medi-Cal Eligibility

Period of Ineligibility Resulting from Gifts of Assets

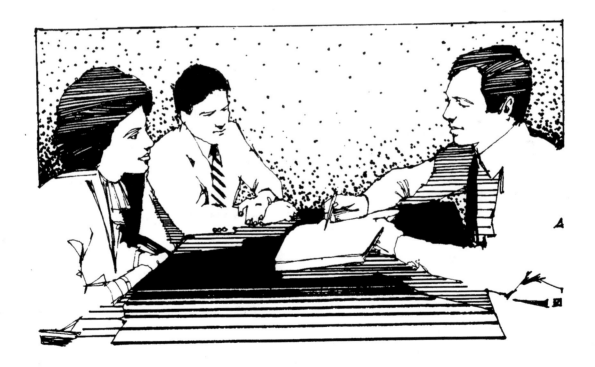

SECTION I

MEDI-CAL ELIGIBILITY RULES FOR MARRIED PERSONS

INTRODUCTION

This chapter explains the Medi-Cal eligibility requirements for an ill spouse who needs nursing home care. It begins with a discussion of the value of the assets owned by a married couple. The chapter also lists and describes the assets that a couple can own which will not be counted toward the Medi-Cal eligibility limits. In addition, it describes the method for determining whether the ill spouse is eligible to receive Medi-Cal benefits. Finally, this chapter discusses how and why Medi-Cal eligibility can be adversely affected by making gifts of assets.

IF MY HUSBAND NEEDS NURSING HOME CARE, CAN HE QUALIFY FOR MEDI-CAL BENEFITS?

An ill spouse may qualify for Medi-Cal benefits if the value of the couple's assets does not exceed $83,960. The value of assets that Medi-Cal categorizes as "exempt" are not counted toward the $83,960 limit.

MY WIFE NEEDS TO ENTER A NURSING HOME. I HAVE SEPARATE PROPERTY FROM A PREVIOUS MARRIAGE. WILL MY SEPARATE PROPERTY BE COUNTED IN DETERMINING MY WIFE'S MEDI-CAL ELIGIBILITY?

Yes. In determining eligibility, Medi-Cal does not distinguish between the couple's community property and separate property. Medi-Cal determines eligibility based on the combined value of assets owned by either or both spouses. Thus, the **combined** value of the couple's separate **and** community property is the basis for determining the Medi-Cal eligibility of the ill spouse.

ARE ALL OF A MARRIED COUPLE'S ASSETS COUNTED IN DETERMINING THE MEDI-CAL ELIGIBILITY OF AN ILL SPOUSE?

Not necessarily. Although Medi-Cal will not distinguish between separate and community property in determining whether an ill spouse is eligible for Medi-Cal, the Medi-Cal Eligibility Worker (EW) will distinguish between assets that are "exempt" from assets that are "non-exempt." If the asset is "exempt," its value is **not** counted toward the $83,960 eligibility limit. If the asset is "non-exempt," then its value will be counted in determining the ill spouse's Medi-Cal eligibility.

WHAT ASSETS ARE "EXEMPT?"

The following are "exempt" assets:

THE PRINCIPAL RESIDENCE

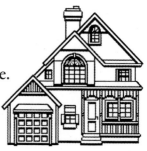

The principal residence is any dwelling that is used as the main residence. It may be a single family home, a mobile home, or an apartment unit. The principal residence is "exempt" **as long as the well spouse continues to remain in the home.**

ONE VEHICLE

Under the Medi-Cal regulations, the value of the principal family vehicle is not counted in determining Medi-Cal eligibility, if it is used for medical purposes such as visiting the ill spouse.

1 Vehicle
(Exempt Asset)
Note: Additional vehicles are countable.

RETIREMENT PLANS

Retirement accounts can include Individual Retirement Accounts (IRAs), 401(k)s, and 403(B) Plans. Under the Medi-Cal regulations, the value of retirement accounts owned by the well spouse is exempt. The value of the ill spouse's retirement accounts is also exempt as long as the ill spouse is receiving periodic distributions from the accounts. A monthly distribution of interest and principal, based on the actuary table of the Social Security Administration, would be sufficient to satisfy this distribution requirement. Caregivers can contact a Financial Planner or Certified Public Accountant (CPA) for information regarding the appropriate monthly distribution amount based the ill spouse's life expectancy.

FIXED ANNUITIES

A fixed annuity is a contract with a life insurance company in which the owner agrees to give funds to the insurance company in exchange for the return of principal and interest over a fixed period of time. Under the Medi-Cal regulations, a fixed annuity is an exempt asset if it satisfies several requirements.

First, the fixed annuity must be irrevocable. As an irrevocable annuity, once it is purchased, the purchaser can never access the principal, except as he or she receives it through distributions. Second, the annuity must make periodic distributions of both interest and principal to the annuity's owner. Periodic distributions include monthly, quarterly or semi-annual distributions. Third, the contract term of the annuity cannot exceed the Medi-Cal applicant's life expectancy, as determined by the Social Security Administration actuary tables. For example, if the patient's life expectancy is ten years, the contract term of the annuity cannot exceed ten years. If the Medi-Cal applicant purchases an annuity contract with a duration that is greater than his or her life expectancy, the annuity purchase could be considered a gift. Under the Medi-Cal regulations, gifts made by either spouse can disqualify the ill spouse from Medi-Cal eligibility. (Disqualifying gifts are discussed later in this chapter).

A life insurance agent or financial planner can provide additional information on fixed annuities.

WHOLE LIFE INSURANCE (up to $1,500 each)

Whole Life Insurance is a form of life insurance that accumulates cash value. The policy stays in force for the lifetime of the insured, unless the policy is canceled or lapses. The whole life insurance policies of each spouse are exempt if the combined face value of each spouse's respective policies is $1,500 or less. If the combined face values of the life insurance owned by either spouse exceed the $1,500 exemption threshold, the cash surrender value is counted toward the couple's $83,960 Medi-Cal eligibility limit.

EXAMPLE

Mr. & Mrs. Smith each own two whole life insurance policies. Mr. Smith's whole life policies have a combined face value of $1,000. Under the Medi-Cal regulations, these policies would be exempt because their combined values do not exceed the $1,500 exemption threshold. However, Mrs. Smith's whole life policies have a combined face value of $3,000. Since the combined values of her whole life policies exceed the $1,500 exemption threshold, the cash surrender value of her policies will be counted toward the couple's $83,960 Medi-Cal eligibility limit.

TERM LIFE INSURANCE
Term Life Insurance is a type of life insurance that is in effect for a specified period. Unlike Whole Life policies, no cash value accumulates with Term Life Insurance. Term Life Insurance is an exempt asset for both spouses.

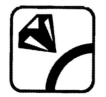

Personal Jewelry
(Exempt Asset)

CLOTHING AND PERSONAL JEWELRY
All personal items, such as clothing and personal jewelry, are exempt.

HOUSEHOLD ITEMS
These include dishes, furniture, clothing, tools, and appliances are exempt. Artwork is exempt as long as it is not held for investment purposes.

PROPERTY USED IN A TRADE OR BUSINESS
Medi-Cal exempts property that is used for a trade or business that is essential for the self-support of either spouse. Such property would include a family business, such as a farm or a retail store. It would also include business inventories, and equipment. However, if a couple owns a rental property, **Medi-Cal will not consider the rental as a business.** Instead, Medi-Cal will view the rental as an investment and, as such, it would **not** fall within the "trade or business" exemption.

BURIAL PLOTS/CRYPTS
Burial plots, Vaults, Crypts, and Caskets are exempt.

BURIAL FUNDS/ PRE-PAID BURIAL PLANS
A Revocable Burial Fund is a fund or account that allows the owner to remove funds at his or her discretion. Under the Medi-Cal regulations,

a Revocable Burial Fund is exempt as long as its value does not exceed $1,500. **Each spouse is allowed a $1,500 Revocable Burial Fund.**

In contrast to a Revocable Burial Fund, an Irrevocable Burial Fund is a fund or account that prohibits the removal of funds unless they are needed for burial purposes. Under the Medi-Cal regulations, Irrevocable Burial Funds are exempt, regardless of their value. As an exempt asset, either spouse can have an Irrevocable Burial Fund and its value will not be counted toward the $83,960 Medi-Cal eligibility limit.

Pre-paid burial plans, including burial insurance, are also exempt. As an exempt asset, either spouse can have a pre-paid burial plan and its value will not be counted toward the $83,960 Medi-Cal eligibility limit.

WHAT ASSETS ARE "NON-EXEMPT?"

In contrast to "exempt" assets, the value of "countable" assets is counted in determining the ill spouse's Medi-Cal eligibility. Another term for "non-exempt" assets is "countable assets." Examples of non-exempt or countable assets include cash, certificates of deposit, mutual funds, stocks, bonds, and rental property.

There are special rules in determining the value of rental property. Under the Medi-Cal regulations, the fair market value is not necessarily the basis for determining the value of the rental property. Rather, Medi-Cal can count the *assessed* value of the rental property less any encumbrance. This is known as the net assessed value. The net assessed value of the rental property is the amount that will be counted toward the $83,960 eligibility limit. Fortunately, for a married couple, the net assessed value is often significantly less than its fair market value. In addition, if the property produces annual income of at least 6 percent of the net assessed value, Medi-Cal will exclude $6,000 from the net assessed value of the property. This is known as the "$6,000/6 percent rule". Essentially, **this rule says that $6,000 will be subtracted from the net assessed value of rental property if the property produces an annual income of at least six percent of the net assessed value.**

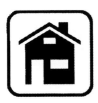

Rental Property
(Countable Asset)

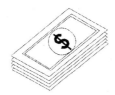

Stocks, Bonds, Mutual Funds
(Countable Assets)

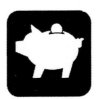

Savings, Cash, CD's
(Countable Assets)

EXAMPLE

John and Mary own a duplex that they rent for $1,000 per month ($12,000 per year),. The rental has a fair market value of $120,000, but it has an assessed value of $30,000. John and Mary owe $10,000 on the duplex. John becomes ill, enters a nursing home, and applies for Medi-Cal benefits.

Medi-Cal will calculate the value of the rental in determining John's Medi-Cal eligibility by using the following formula:

Net Assessed Value
– $6,000 exemption

**Value Counted Toward
Medi-Cal Eligibility**

Step One: First, Medi-Cal will calculate the net assessed value of the property. This is accomplished by taking the assessed value of the property ($30,000) and subtracting the encumbrance ($10,000). Thus, the net assessed value is $20,000.

Step Two: Second, Medi-Cal will subtract $6,000 from the $20,000 net assessed value. Medi-cal does this because, in this example, the rental produces annual income which is at least **6 percent of the net assessed value ($1,200)** –thus qualifying it for the $6,000 exclusion under the Medi-Cal regulations. Therefore, Medi-Cal will value the rental at $14,000 for the purpose of determining John's Medi-Cal eligibility.

In summary, the calculation would look like this:

Step One: Determine Net Assessed Value:	$30,000
	– $10,000
	$20,000
Step Two: Subtract $6,000 from the net assessed value:	– $6,000
Value Counted toward Medi-Cal eligibility:	**$14,000**

HOW CAN I DETERMINE IF MY SPOUSE IS ELIGIBLE FOR MEDI-CAL BENEFITS?

To make this determination, follow the same procedure used by Medi-Cal:

> **Step One:** *List* the *types* and *values* of the couple's assets including all separate and community property owned by both spouses.

> **Step Two:** *Categorize* the assets as "exempt" or "non-exempt".

> **Step Three:** *Add* the total value of the non-exempt assets.

In order for the ill spouse to be eligible for Medi-Cal benefits, the combined value of the couple's non-exempt assets must fall within the $83,960 eligibility limit for married persons. Medi-Cal determines eligibility based on the combined value of assets owned by either or both spouses.

EXAMPLE

John and Mary have been married for fifty years. John and Mary have a $20,000 Certificate of Deposit, which they own jointly. Mary has $25,000 in savings in her name only. John and Mary's home, owned free and clear, is worth $150,000. John and Mary also own a car worth $5,000. John enters into a nursing home.

The following is the method for determining whether John is eligible for Medi-Cal benefits

Step One: List the type and value of assets owned by either or both spouses.

Type	Spouse	Value
Home	(John + Mary)	$150,000
Certificates of Deposit	(John + Mary)	$20,000
Savings	(Mary)	$25,000
Car	(John + Mary)	$5,000

Step Two: Categorize the asset as "exempt or non-exempt".

Type	Category	Value
Home	***Exempt***	$150,000
Certificates of Deposit	Non-Exempt	$20,000
Savings	Non-Exempt	$25,000
Car	***Exempt***	$5,000

Step Three: Add the total value of the non-exempt assets.

Type	Category	Value
Certificates of Deposit	Non-Exempt	$20,000
Savings	Non-Exempt	$25,000
		$20,000
		+ $25,000
Total Value of Non-Exempt Assets		**$45,000**

Thus, under the Medi-Cal regulations, John will qualify for Medi-Cal benefits because the value of his non-exempt assets is within the Medi-Cal eligibility limit of $83,960 for a married person.

MY WIFE IS NOT ELIGIBLE FOR MEDI-CAL BENEFITS BECAUSE THE VALUE OF OUR NON-EXEMPT ASSETS EXCEEDS THE ELIGIBILITY LIMIT. IF WE GIVE AWAY OUR EXCESS ASSETS, WILL SHE BECOME ELIGIBLE FOR MEDI-CAL BENEFITS?

Making gifts of assets will not automatically make the ill spouse eligible for Medi-Cal benefits. In fact, giving away assets may automatically make the ill spouse **ineligible** for Medi-Cal benefits for a period of time, even though the value of their non-exempt assets falls within the $83,960 Medi-Cal eligibility limit.

There is a reason for this penalty. Medi-Cal does not want people to give away assets (e.g., make gifts) that could have been used to pay for the cost of their care. Consequently, Medi-Cal may penalize the Medi-Cal applicant if the couple transfers an asset for less than fair market value within 30 months of applying for Medi-Cal benefits. The penalty for making such a gift is the imposition of a "period of ineligibility" for Medi-Cal benefits. Under this rule, if a period of ineligibility is in effect, the ill spouse cannot receive Medi-Cal benefits **even if the value of their non-exempt assets falls within the Medi-Cal eligibility limits.**

EXAMPLE

John and Mary are married. On May 1, they had combined non-exempt assets of $100,000. On June 1, John and Mary gave $25,000 to their son, Bill, for a down payment on a home. On July 1, Mary became ill, entered a nursing home, and applied for Medi-Cal benefits. Although the value of John and Mary's non-exempt assets now falls within the $83,960 Medi-Cal eligibility limit, Mary is under a period of ineligibility because of the $25,000 gift. Consequently, she will not receive Medi-Cal benefits as long as the period of ineligibility remains in effect.

WHAT IF MY WIFE AND I SELL AN ASSET TO OUR CHILDREN AT A SUBSTANTIAL DISCOUNT. WILL THIS "SALE" CAUSE A PERIOD OF INELIGIBILITY?

Under the Medi-Cal rules, a gift is actually a transfer of assets for less than fair market value. Consequently, if an asset is sold at a discount to its fair market value, Medi-Cal can impose a period of ineligibility based on the the difference between the fair market value of the property and the actual amount received in exchange for it.

EXAMPLE

John and Mary own a recreational vehicle (RV) that is worth $10,000. If John and Mary "sold" the RV to their son Bill for $500, Medi-Cal would consider this "sale" as a gift of $9500 since it was sold for $9500 less than its fair market value. Thus, this "sale" of the RV would result in a period of ineligibility for either John or Mary.

CAN EACH SPOUSE GIVE AWAY $10,000 A YEAR WITHOUT CAUSING A PERIOD OF INELIGIBILITY?

There is a rule of law that allows each spouse to make a gift of up to $10,000 per year without incurring federal gift taxes. However, this rule does not apply to Medi-Cal. Cash gifts of $10,000 by either spouse can result in a period of ineligibility for Medi-Cal.

IF A COUPLE GIVES AWAY AN ASSET, HOW LONG DOES A PERIOD OF INELIGIBILITY REMAIN IN EFFECT?

When a gift of an asset is made by either spouse, the period of ineligibility will begin on that date, and its duration will depend upon the value of the gift. Basically, the period of ineligibility will be equal to the number of months of nursing home care that could have been paid for by the asset that was gifted. However, under current Medi-Cal regulations, the maximum duration of the period of ineligibility for any single gift will be 30 months.†

† In 1993, rules enacted by Congress allow Medi-Cal to eliminate the 30 month "cap" on the period of ineligibility. As of the date of the publication of this book, Medi-Cal still adheres to the 30 month maximum period of ineligibility rule. However, this could change at any time. Please consult an elder law attorney for the most current rules.

HOW DOES MEDI-CAL CALCULATE THE DURATION OF THE PERIOD OF INELIGIBILITY?

Basically, Medi-Cal calculates the duration of the period of ineligibility by dividing the value of the asset gifted by the average monthly cost of nursing home care in California. (In 1999, the average cost of nursing home care is $3,882 per month). Thus, calculating the duration of the period of ineligibility requires two steps:

Step One: Determine the amount of the gift. (Note: if there are multiple gifts, add the amounts of these gifts).

Step Two: Divide the amount of the gift by $3,882 (the average private pay rate per month for nursing home care).

EXAMPLE

John and Mary, a married couple, have non-exempt assets valued at $100,000. On June 1, they gave their son $25,000 for a down payment on a house. The following month, Mary became ill, entered a nursing home, and applied for Medi-Cal benefits. She is under a period of ineligibility for Medi-Cal benefits as a result of the gift.

The duration of the period of ineligibility is determined as follows:

Step One: Determine the amount of the gift: $25,000

Step Two: Divide the amount of the gift by $3,882 per month (the average private pay rate per month for nursing home care):

$$\begin{array}{r} \$25,000 \\ \div \quad \$3,882 \text{ per month} \\ \hline \textbf{6.4 months} \end{array}$$

Mary is under a period of ineligibility for seven months (fractions are disregarded). Since the period of ineligibility begins when the gift is made, Mary will be ineligible for Medi-Cal from June 1 until January 1 of the following year.

HOW FAR BACK DOES MEDI-CAL LOOK TO DETERMINE WHETHER A GIFT WOULD CAUSE A PERIOD OF INELIGIBILITY?

Medi-Cal is not concerned with gifts the couple may have made many years ago. When the ill spouse applies for Medi-Cal benefits, Medi-Cal will only look back 30 months from the date of application to determine if the couple made any gifts. This is known as the "30-month look back" rule. Thus, when the ill spouse applies for Medi-Cal benefits, Medi-Cal will ask on the application whether the couple has made a gift of an asset within the last 30 months. If there have been no gifts within the 30-month time frame, then then there will be no period of ineligibility.

EXAMPLE

In 1993, John and Mary, a married couple, gave their son and daughter-in-law a gift of $25,000 to help them purchase their first home. In 1999, Mary entered a nursing home and applied for Medi-Cal benefits. Medi-Cal will only look back 30-months from the date of application for Medi-Cal benefits to determine whether the couple made a gift of assets that would cause a period of ineligibility. Since this gift occurred five years before Mary applied for Medi-Cal, which is well beyond the 30-month look back period, Mary will not subject to a period of ineligibility period.†

DO ALL GIFTS MADE WITHIN THE 30-MONTH LOOK BACK PERIOD CAUSE A PERIOD OF INELIGIBILITY?

No. Medi-Cal allows the gifting of some assets without imposing a period of ineligibility. Such gifts are called "exempt transfers". Whether a gift can be categorized as an "exempt transfer" depends on the type, as well as the recipient, of the asset.

The following are examples of exempt transfers:

1) Gifts between spouses;
2) A gift of the home to an adult child who is permanently and totally disabled;
3) A gift of the home to a sibling with an equity interest in the home and who resided in the home at least one year prior to the ill person's entry into the nursing home; and
4) A gift of the home to an adult child who resided at least two years in the home and by providing care, he or she delayed the institutionalization of their parent.

Section I: SUMMARY

1. An ill spouse could qualify for Medi-Cal if the value of the couple's assets does not exceed $83,960. In determining Medi-Cal eligibility, the assets of the ill person are categorized as either "exempt" or "exempt." If the asset is "exempt," its value is **not counted** toward the $83,960 eligibility limit. If the asset is "non-exempt," then its value is counted in determining the ill spouse's Medi-Cal eligibility.

2. The principal residence of the couple is exempt as long as the well spouse continues to live in the home. Other examples of exempt assets include one vehicle, household goods, burial plots, irrevocable burial funds. Under certain conditions, retirement accounts, annuities, and life insurance are also exempt.

3. Non-exempt assets include cash, stocks, bonds, mutual funds, and rental property. In determining eligibility, Medi-Cal can count the rental property's net assessed value towards the $83,960 eligibility limit. The net assessed value is the actual assessed value of the property minus any encumbrances.

4. In addition, if the rental property produces annual income that is at least 6 percent of the net assessed value, Medi-Cal will exclude

†Recent changes in the law allow Medi-Cal to extend this 30 month look back period to 36 months. If a gift is made from a living trust, the new rules authorize Medi-Cal to look back 60 months from the date of application. However, as of the publication of this book, Medi-Cal continues to only look back 30 months for any gifts of assets. Please consult an attorney for the most current Medi-Cal rules.

$6,000 from the net assessed value of the property. This is known as the "$6,000/6 percent rule".

5. If the property meets this income producing requirement, the formula for calculating the non-exempt (countable) value of the rental property would be as follows:

$$\begin{array}{r} \text{Net Assessed Value} \\ -\quad \text{\$6,000 exemption} \\ \hline \textbf{Value Counted Toward} \\ \textbf{Medi-Cal Eligibility} \end{array}$$

6. The step-by-step method of determining whether your loved one is eligible for Medi-Cal is as follows:

   Step One: List the **type** and **value** of the couple's assets.

   Step Two: Categorize the assets as "exempt" or "non-exempt."

   Step Three: Add the total value of the **non-exempt** assets.

7. Giving away assets could make the ill spouse **ineligible** for Medi-Cal benefits for a period of time, even if the value of her non-exempt assets falls within the $83,960 Medi-Cal eligibility limit subsequent to the gift.

8. The period of ineligibility begins on the date that the gift was made. Determining the duration of the period of ineligibility requires the following:

   Step One: Calculate the amount of the gift.

   Step Two: Divide the amount of the gift by $3,882 per month (the Average Private pay rate per month for nursing home care)

9. Under the 30 month "look back period," Medi-Cal will not inquire about gifts made beyond 30 months from the date of application. Thus, gifts made beyond 30 months from the date of application for Medi-Cal will not result a period of ineligibility.

10. The couple can make some gifts, even within the 30-month look back period, and Medi-Cal will not impose a period of ineligibility. These types of gifts are known as "exempt transfers." A gift between spouses is an example of an exempt transfer.

SECTION II

MEDI-CAL ELIGIBILITY RULES FOR SINGLE PERSONS

IF MY LOVED ONE NEEDS TO ENTER A NURSING HOME, WHAT IS THE MAXIMUM AMOUNT OF ASSETS SHE CAN OWN AND QUALIFY FOR MEDI-CAL BENEFITS?

In order to qualify for Medi-Cal benefits, the value of your loved one's combined assets cannot exceed $2,000. However, in determining whether your loved one is eligible for Medi-Cal benefits, the Medi-Cal Eligibility Worker (EW) will divide the assets into two categories: "exempt" and "non-exempt." If the asset is "exempt," its value **will not be counted** toward the $2,000 eligibility limit. If the asset is "non-exempt," then its value will be counted in determining your loved one's Medi-Cal eligibility.

WHAT ASSETS ARE "EXEMPT"?

The following are "exempt" assets:

THE PRINCIPAL RESIDENCE

The principal residence is any dwelling that is used as the main residence. It may be a single family home, a mobile home, or an apartment unit. The principal residence is an exempt asset as long **as the person applying for Medi-Cal benefits intends to return to the home.** This "intent to return home" requirement is subjective. This means that the intent to return home requirement is satisfied if, in the patient's mind, he or she intends to return home. This requirement can even be satisfied by persons suffering from advanced dementia. The likelihood that the ill person will return home is irrelevant. The main purpose of this rule is to provide nursing home patients with hope that one day they will return home. Indeed, it is this hope that keeps many nursing home patients alive. Anyone applying for Medi-Cal benefits on behalf of their loved one has the authority to place a checkmark in the box asking if the Medi-Cal applicant intends to return home. Checking this box "yes" can preserve the home for the ill person while she is receiving Medi-Cal benefits.

ONE VEHICLE

Under the Medi-Cal regulations, the value of the principal family vehicle is not counted in determining Medi-Cal eligibility.

1 Vehicle
(Exempt Asset)
Note: Additional vehicles are countable.

RETIREMENT PLANS

Under the Medi-Cal regulations, the value of Individual Retirement Accounts (IRAs), 401(k)s, and 403(B) retirement plans is not counted in determining Medi-Cal eligibility as long as the Medi-Cal applicant is receiving a periodic distribution from the account. A monthly distribution of interest and principal, made in accordance with the patient's life expectancy as determined by the actuary tables of the Social Security Administration, would be sufficient to satisfy this distribution requirement. Caregivers can contact a Financial Planner or Certified Public Accountant (CPA) for information regarding the appropriate monthly distribution amount based on your loved one's life expectancy.

FIXED ANNUITIES

An annuity is a contract with a life insurance company in which the owner agrees to give funds to the insurance company in exchange for the return of principal and interest over a fixed period of time. Under the Medi-Cal regulations, a fixed annuity is an exempt asset if it satisfies three requirements.

First, it must by irrevocable. As an irrevocable annuity, once it is purchased, the purchaser can never access the principal, except as he or she receives it through distributions. Second, the annuity must make periodic distributions of both interest and principal to the annuity's owner. Periodic distributions include monthly, quarterly or semi-annual distributions. Third, the contract term of the annuity cannot exceed the Medi-Cal applicant's life expectancy, as determined by the Social Security Administration actuary tables. For example, if the patient's life expectancy is ten years, the contract term of the annuity cannot exceed ten years. If the Medi-Cal applicant purchases an annuity contract in excess of his or her life expectancy, the annuity purchase could be considered a gift, which would disqualify him or her for Medi-Cal benefits. (Disqualifying gifts are discussed later in this chapter). You should consult a financial planner or CPA for the appropriate distribution amounts based on life expectancy of the retirement account's owner. In addition, a life insurance agent or financial planner can provide you with additional information regarding fixed annuities.

WHOLE LIFE INSURANCE (up to $1,500)

Whole Life Insurance is a form of life insurance that accumulates cash value. The policy stays in force for the lifetime of the insured, unless the policy is canceled or lapses. In determining eligibility, Medi-Cal combines the face value of all Whole Life Insurance policies owned by the applicant. If the combined face values are $1,500 or less, the Whole Life Insurance is exempt. However, if the combined face values of the life insurance exceed $1,500, the cash surrender value is counted toward the $2,000 Medi-Cal eligibility limit.

EXAMPLE

Mrs. Smith, a widow, is in a nursing home and applies for Medi-Cal benefits. She owns two whole life insurance policies which have a combined face value of $5,000. Since the combined values of her whole life policies exceed the $1,500 exemption threshold, the cash surrender value of her policies will be counted toward the $2,000 Medi-Cal eligibility limit.

TERM LIFE INSURANCE

Term Life Insurance is a type of life insurance that is in effect for a specified period. Unlike Whole Life policies, no cash value accumulates with Term Life Insurance. The face value of a Term Life Insurance policy is exempt.

PERSONAL JEWELRY AND CLOTHING

Engagement rings, wedding rings, and heirlooms are exempt assets. All other jewelry and other personal items such as clothing are exempt if the combined net value of these items is less than $100.

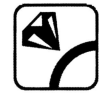

Personal Jewelry
(Exempt Asset)

HOUSEHOLD ITEMS

These include dishes, furniture, clothing, tools, and appliances. These are all exempt assets. Artwork is exempt as long as it is not held for investment purposes.

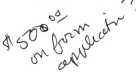

PROPERTY USED IN A TRADE OR BUSINESS

Medi-Cal exempts property that is used for a trade or business that is essential for the self-support of the ill person. Such property would include a family business, such as a farm or a retail store. It would also include business inventories and equipment. However, if the ill person owns rental property, **Medi-Cal will not consider the rental as a business.** Instead, Medi-Cal will view the rental as an investment and, as such, it would **not** fall within the "trade or business" exemption.

BURIAL PLOTS/CRYPTS

Burial plots, vaults, crypts, and caskets are all exempt.

PRE-PAID BURIAL PLANS/BURIAL FUNDS

A Revocable Burial Fund is an account that allows the owner to remove funds at his or her discretion. Under the Medi-Cal regulations, such an account or fund is an exempt asset if its value does not exceed $1,500.

In contrast to a Revocable Burial Fund, an Irrevocable Burial Fund is an account or fund that prohibits the removal of funds unless they are needed for burial purposes. Under the Medi-Cal regulations, an Irrevocable Burial Fund is an exempt asset, regardless of its value. A pre-paid burial plan, including burial insurance, is exempt.

WHAT ASSETS ARE "NON-EXEMPT?"

In contrast to "exempt" assets, the value of "non-exempt" assets is counted in determining the ill person's Medi-Cal eligibility. Examples of countable assets, otherwise known as "non-exempt assets" include cash, certificates of

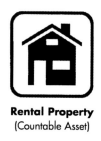

Rental Property
(Countable Asset)

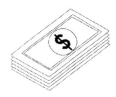

**Stocks, Bonds,
Mutual Funds**
(Countable Assets)

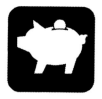

**Savings,
Cash,
CD's**
(Countable Assets)

deposit, mutual funds, stocks, bonds, and rental property. However, there are special rules in determining the value of rental property.

Under the Medi-Cal regulations, the fair market value is not necessarily the basis for determining the value of the property. Rather, Medi-Cal can count the *assessed* value of the rental property minus any encumbrances. This is known as the net assessed value. Thus, Medi-Cal counts the net assessed value toward the $2,000 eligibility limit. Fortunately for most Medi-Cal applicants, the net assessed value is often significantly less than its fair market value. In addition, **if the property produces annual income that is at least 6 percent of the net assessed value,** Medi-Cal will exclude $6,000 from the net assessed value of the property. This is known as the "$6,000/6 percent rule". **This rule says that $6,000 will be subtracted from the net assessed value of rental property if the property produces an annual income of at least 6 percent of the net assessed value.**

EXAMPLE

John, a widower, owns a home and a duplex that he rents for $1,000 per month. The property has a fair market value of $120,000, but it has an assessed value of $30,000. John owes $10,000 on the duplex. John recently entered a nursing home and applied for Medi-Cal benefits.

The value of John's rental property will be determined as follows:

Net Assessed Value
− $6,000 exemption
_____
**Value Counted Toward
Medi-Cal Eligibility**

Step One: First, Medi-Cal will calculate the net assessed value of the property. This is accomplished by taking the assessed value of the property ($30,000) and subtracting the encumbrance ($10,000). Thus, the net assessed value is $20,000.

Step Two: Second, Medi-Cal will subtract $6,000 from the $20,000 net assessed value. Medi-Cal will deduct $6,000 from the net assessed value because, in this example, the rental produces annual income which is at least **6 percent of the net assessed value ($1200 per year)** –thus qualifying it for the $6,000 exclusion under the Medi-Cal regulations. Thus, Medi-Cal will value the rental at $14,000 for the purpose of determining John's Medi-Cal eligibility.

In summary, the calculation would look like this:

Step One: Determine Net Assessed Value:	$30,000
	– $10,000
	$20,000
Step Two: Subtract $6,000 from the net assessed value:	– $6,000
Value Counted toward Medi-Cal eligibility:	$14,000

I WOULD LIKE TO RENT MY LOVED ONE'S RESIDENCE WHILE HE IS IN THE NURSING HOME. DOES THE RESIDENCE BECOME NON-EXEMPT ONCE IT'S RENTED?

Renting the principal residence while your loved one is in the nursing home does not transform the residence into non-exempt rental property. The principal residence continues to be an exempt asset, as long as your loved one intends to return home.

HOW CAN I DETERMINE IF MY LOVED ONE IS ELIGIBLE FOR MEDI-CAL BENEFITS?

To make this determination, follow the same procedure used by Medi-Cal:

Step One: List the **type** and **value** of your loved one's assets (e.g., Savings—$10,000).

Step Two: Categorize the assets as "exempt" or "non-exempt".

Step Three: Add the total value of the non-exempt assets.

EXAMPLE

The following is an example of how the Medi-Cal eligibility rules work for a single person: Elizabeth is a widow. She owns her home, free and clear, which is worth approximately 120,000.

She has $1,000 in a checking account, and $500 in a savings account. She owns a 1984 Ford Escort that is worth $2,000. Finally, she has a paid-up burial plan worth $4,000. Elizabeth enters into a nursing home, but she intends to return home. She applies for Medi-Cal benefits. The Medi-Cal eligibility limit for a single person in 1999 is $2,000.

Elizabeth's Medi-Cal eligibility can be determined as follows:

Step One: List the **type** and **value** of Elizabeth's assets.

Type	Value
Home	$120,000
Checking Account	$1,000
Savings	$500
Car	$2,000
Burial Plan	$4,000

Step Two: Categorize the asset as "exempt or non-exempt".

Type	Category	Value
Home	***Exempt***	$120,000
Checking Account	Non-Exempt	$1,000
Savings	Non-Exempt	$500
Car	**Exempt***	$2,000
Burial Plan	**Exempt***	$4,000

Step Three: Add the total value of the **non-exempt** assets.

Type	Category	Value
Checking Account	**Non-Exempt**	**$1,000**
Savings	**Non-Exempt**	**$500**
		$1,000
		+ $500
Total Value of Non-Exempt Assets		**$1,500**

Thus, under the Medi-Cal regulations, Elizabeth will qualify for Medi-Cal benefits **because the value of her non-exempt (countable) assets is within the Medi-Cal eligibility limit of $2,000 for a single person.**

MY LOVED ONE IS NOT ELIGIBLE FOR MEDI-CAL BENEFITS BECAUSE THE VALUE OF HER NON-EXEMPT ASSETS EXCEEDS THE $2,000 ELIGIBILITY LIMIT. CAN SHE BECOME ELIGIBLE FOR MEDI-CAL BENEFITS IF SHE GIVES AWAY HER ASSETS?

Making gifts of assets will not automatically make your loved one eligible for Medi-Cal benefits. In fact, giving away assets could make your loved one **ineligible** for Medi-Cal benefits for a period of time, even if the value of her non-exempt assets falls within the $2,000 Medi-Cal eligibility limit.

There is a reason for this penalty. Medi-Cal does not want people to give away assets (e.g., make gifts) that could have been used to pay for the cost of their care. Consequently, Medi-Cal may penalize the Medi-Cal applicant if he or she transfers an asset for less than fair market value within 30 months of applying for Medi-Cal benefits. The penalty for making such a gift is the imposition of a "period of ineligibility" for Medi-Cal benefits. If a period of ineligibility is in effect, your loved one cannot receive Medi-Cal benefits **even if the value of his or her non-exempt assets falls within the Medi-Cal eligibility limit.**

EXAMPLE

Mary is a widow. On May 1, she had non-exempt (countable) assets valued at $22,000. On June 1, she gave her two grandchildren $10,000 each. On July 1, Mary became ill, entered a nursing home, and applied for Medi-Cal benefits. At the time of application, Mary had non-exempt assets valued at $2,000. **Mary is NOT eligible for Medi-Cal benefits**

Although the value of Mary's non-exempt (countable) assets falls within the Medi-Cal eligibility limit of $2,000, Mary is under a period of ineligibility as a result of the $20,000 cash gift made to her grandchildren.

WHAT IF MY LOVED ONE SELLS AN ASSET AT A SUBSTANTIAL DISCOUNT TO ITS FAIR MARKET VALUE. WILL THIS "SALE" CAUSE A PERIOD OF INELIGIBILITY?

Under the Medi-Cal rules, a gift is actually a transfer of assets for less than fair market value. Consequently, if an asset is sold at a discount to its fair market value, Medi-Cal can impose a period of ineligibility based on the the difference between the fair market value of the property and the actual amount received in exchange for it.

EXAMPLE

Mary, a widow, owns a recreational vehicle (RV) that is worth $10,000. If Mary "sold" the RV to her son Bill for $500, Medi-Cal would consider this "sale" as a gift of $9500 since it was sold for $9500 less than its fair market value. Thus, this "sale" of the RV would result in a period of ineligibility for Mary.

CAN MY LOVED ONE GIVE AWAY $10,000 A YEAR WITHOUT CAUSING A PERIOD OF INELIGIBILITY?

There is a rule of law that allows an individual to make a gift of up to $10,000 without incurring federal gift taxes. However, this rule has nothing to do with Medi-Cal. Cash gifts of $10,000 can result in a period of ineligibility for Medi-Cal.

IF MY LOVED ONE GIVES AWAY ASSETS, HOW LONG DOES THE PERIOD OF INELIGIBILITY FOR MEDI-CAL BENEFITS REMAIN IN EFFECT?

When a gift of an asset is made, the period of ineligibility will begin on that date, and its duration will depend upon the value of the gift. Basically, the period of ineligibility will be equal to the number of months of nursing home care that could have been paid for by the asset that was gifted. However, under current Medi-Cal regulations, the maximum duration of the period of ineligibility for any single gift will be 30 months.†

†In 1993, rules enacted by Congress allow Medi-Cal to eliminate the 30 month "cap" on the period of ineligibility. As of the date of the publication of this book, Medi-Cal still adheres to the 30 month maximum period of ineligibility rule. However, this could change at any time. Please consult an elder law attorney for the most current rules.

HOW DOES MEDI-CAL CALCULATE THE DURATION OF THE PERIOD OF INELIGIBILITY?

Basically, Medi-Cal calculates the duration of the period of ineligibility by dividing the value of the asset gifted by the average monthly cost of nursing home care in California. (In 1999, the average cost of nursing home care is $3,882 per month).

EXAMPLE

Mary is a widow. On May 1, she had non-exempt assets valued at $22,000. On June 1, she gave her son $20,000. On July 1, Mary became ill, entered a nursing home, and applied for Medi-Cal benefits. Because of the gift, at the time of application, Mary only had $2,000 in non-exempt assets.

The duration of the period of ineligibility is calculated as follows

Step One: Determine the amount of the gift

Mary gave away $20,000

Step Two: Divide the amount of the gift by $3,882 per month (the Average Private pay rate per month for nursing home care):

$20,000
÷ $3,882 per month
5.1 months

MARY IS UNDER A PERIOD OF INELIGIBILITY FOR FIVE MONTHS (fractions are disregarded). Under the Medi-Cal regulations, the period of ineligibility begins on the date the gift was made—in this case, June 1. **Thus, Mary will not be eligible for Medi-Cal benefits until November 1.**

HOW FAR BACK DOES MEDI-CAL LOOK TO DETERMINE WHETHER MY LOVED ONE MADE A GIFT THAT WOULD RESULT IN A PERIOD OF INELIGIBILITY?

Medi-Cal is not concerned with gifts your loved one may have made many years ago. When the ill person applies for Medi-Cal benefits, Medi-Cal will only look back 30 months from the date of application to determine if the he or she made any gifts. This is known as the "30-month look back" rule. Thus, when the ill person applies for Medi-Cal benefits, Medi-Cal will ask on the application whether he or she has made any gifts of assets within the last 30 months. If there have been no gifts within the 30 month time frame, then then there will be no period of ineligibility.

EXAMPLE

In 1993, Albert, a widower, gave $25,000 to his son to help him purchase his first home. In 1999, Albert entered into a nursing home and applied for Medi-Cal benefits. Medi-Cal will look back only 30 months from the date Albert applies for Medi-Cal benefits to determine if he has made a gift of assets which would cause a period of ineligibility. In this example, Medi-Cal will not be concerned about the $25,000 gift because it occurred five years before Albert applied for Medi-Cal, which is well beyond the 30-month look back period.†

†Recent changes in the law allow Medi-Cal to extend this 30 month look back period to 36-months. If a gift is made from a living trust, the new rules authorize Medi-Cal to look back 60 months from the date of application. However, as of the publication of this book, Medi-Cal continues to only look back 30 months for any gifts of assets. Please consult an attorney for the most current Medi-Cal rules.

DO ALL GIFTS MADE WITHIN THE 30-MONTH LOOK BACK PERIOD CAUSE A PERIOD OF INELIGIBILITY?

No. Medi-Cal allows the gifting of some assets without imposing a period of ineligibility. These types of gifts are called "exempt transfers." Whether the gift constitutes an "exempt transfer" depends on the type, as well as the recipient, of the asset.

The following are examples of "exempt" transfers that are relevant to single persons:

1) The transfer of the home to an adult child who is blind or who is permanently and totally disabled;

2) The transfer of the home to a sibling with an equity interest in the home and who resided in the home at least one year prior to the ill person's entry into the nursing home and

3) The transfer of the home to an adult child who resided at least two years in the home and by providing care, he or she delayed the institutionalization of his or her parent.

Section II: SUMMARY

1. An ill person could qualify for Medi-Cal if the value of his or her assets does not exceed $2,000. In determining Medi-Cal eligibility, the assets of the ill person are categorized as either "exempt" or "exempt." If the asset is "exempt," its value is **not counted** toward the $2,000 eligibility limit. If the asset is "non-exempt," then its value is counted in determining your loved one's Medi-Cal eligibility.

2. The principal residence of the ill person is exempt as long as he or she intends to return home. The intent to return home requirement is subjective; it depends upon the actual intent of the ill person to return home, not the likelihood that he or she will return home. Other examples of exempt assets include one vehicle, household goods, burial plots, irrevocable burial funds. Under certain conditions, retirement accounts, annuities, and life insurance are also exempt.

3. Non-exempt assets include cash, stocks, bonds, mutual funds, and rental property. In determining eligibility, Medi-Cal will count the net assessed value of the rental property. The net assessed value is the actual assessed value of the property minus any encumbrances.

4. In addition, if the rental property produces annual income that is at least 6 percent of the net assessed value, Medi-Cal will exclude $6,000 from the net assessed value of the property. This is known as the "$6,000/6 percent rule".

5. If the property meets this income producing requirement, the formula for calculating the non-exempt (countable) value of the rental property would be as follows:

$$
\begin{array}{r}
\text{Net Assessed Value} \\
-\quad \$6{,}000 \text{ exclusion} \\
\hline
\textbf{Value Counted Toward} \\
\textbf{Medi-Cal Eligibility}
\end{array}
$$

6. The step-by-step method of determining whether your loved one is eligible for Medi-Cal is as follows:

   Step One: List the **type** and **value** of your loved one's assets.

   Step Two: Categorize the assets as "exempt" or "non-exempt".

   Step Three: Add the total value of the non-exempt assets.

7. Giving away assets could make your loved one **ineligible** for Medi-Cal benefits for a period of time, even if the value of her non-exempt assets falls within the $2,000 Medi-Cal eligibility limit.

8. The period of ineligibility begins on the date that the gift was made. Determining the duration of the period of ineligibility requires the following:

   Step One: Determine the amount of the gift.

   Step Two: Divide the amount of the gift by $3,882 per month (the average private pay rate per month for nursing home care).

9. Under the 30 month "look back period," Medi-Cal will not inquire about gifts made beyond 30 months from the date of application. Thus, gifts made beyond 30 months from the date of application for Medi-Cal will not result a period of ineligibility.

10. The Medi-Cal applicant can make some gifts, even within the 30 month look back period, and Medi-Cal will not impose a period of ineligibility. These types of gifts are known as "exempt transfers." A gift of the home to an adult disabled child is an example of an exempt transfer.

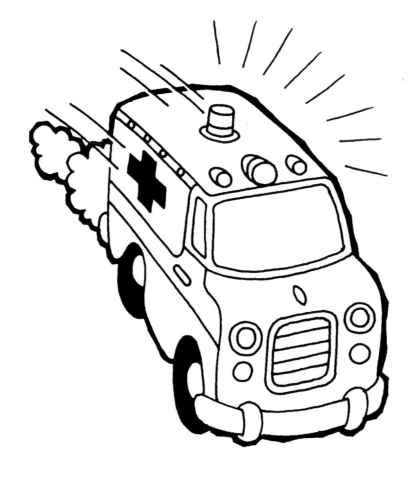

CHAPTER 3

ASSET PROTECTION STRATEGIES

This chapter covers the following:

Strategies for protecting cash and/or securities.

Strategies for protecting rental property.

A Strategy for protecting retirement accounts.

A Strategy for protecting life insurance.

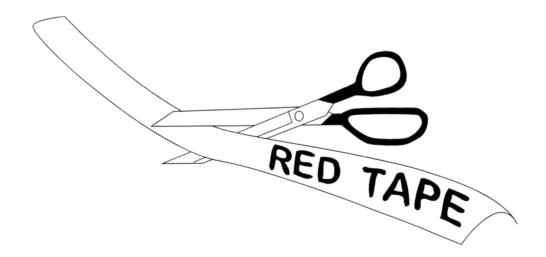

SECTION I

ASSET PROTECTION STRATEGIES FOR MARRIED PERSONS

WHAT HAPPENS IF A MARRIED COUPLE HAS ASSETS WHICH EXCEED THE MEDI-CAL ELIGIBILITY LIMIT WHEN AN ILL SPOUSE APPLIES FOR MEDI-CAL BENEFITS?

If a married couple has assets in excess of the Medi-Cal eligibility limit, the ill spouse is ineligible to receive Medi-Cal benefits. In this situation, the State prefers that the couple pay the nursing home for the cost of the ill spouse's care until the couple has spent down to the $83,960 Medi-Cal eligibility limit. At that time, the ill spouse may become eligible for Medi-Cal benefits.

WHAT IS THE DANGER OF SPENDING DOWN TO THE ELIGIBILITY LIMIT?

The potential danger of the "spend down" option is that well spouse may not be left with sufficient assets to meet his or her financial, personal, and health care needs. In addition, since Medi-Cal does not pay every health care cost, there may be medical procedures or equipment which the ill spouse needs that are not covered by Medi-Cal. However, if they have spent down to the Medi-Cal eligibility limit, then the couple may not have sufficient assets to pay for these needed medical procedures or equipment.

ARE THERE ANY ALTERNATIVES TO SPENDING DOWN TO THE MEDI-CAL ELIGIBILITY LIMIT?

There are various asset protection strategies that serve as alternatives to the traditional "spend down" option. The following are some proven strategies that can effectively protect assets for the well spouse, while enabling the ill spouse to become Medi-Cal eligible. Either one strategy, or a combination of the strategies listed, may be useful. However, the appropriateness of each asset protection strategy depends on the type and nature of the asset to be protected. For example, strategies to protect cash differ from strategies to protect real estate.

ASSET PROTECTION STRATEGIES
PROTECTION OF CASH/SECURITIES

There are five basic strategies that can be used to protect the couple's excess cash and or securities:

- **A. CONVERT CASH INTO EXEMPT ASSETS.**
- **B. PURCHASE AN IRREVOCABLE ANNUITY IN THE NAME OF THE WELL SPOUSE.**
- **C. TRANSFER ASSETS OUT OF THE COUPLE'S ESTATE.**
- **D. PAY OFF DEBTS (EXCEPT UNPAID MEDICAL BILLS).**
- **E. OBTAIN A COURT ORDER.**

STRATEGY A

CONVERT CASH INTO EXEMPT ASSETS

A married couple can convert its excess cash into exempt assets. This is accomplished by using cash assets to purchase exempt assets. For example, if the non-exempt assets exceed the Medi-Cal eligibility limit but the couple have a mortgage, the excess cash can be used to pay off the mortgage. The same principle applies to home repairs, remodeling the home, paying attorney's fees, purchasing personal jewelry and household items, purchasing burial plots, and establishing burial funds.

Another example is that each spouse can purchase revocable and irrevocable burial funds. A revocable burial fund is a separate trust fund or savings account in which the funds are used to pay for burial expenses. One can place funds in a revocable burial fund and later terminate the fund if he or she desires. Monies placed in a revocable burial fund will not be counted in determining the ill spouse's Medi-Cal eligibility if the value of the fund does not exceed $1,500.

Each spouse can also purchase an irrevocable burial fund. Irrevocable burial funds are trust funds that are used for burial expenses. However, once the married person places the funds in the account, he or she cannot later terminate the account. *Unlike revocable burial funds, there is no limit on the amount each of the spouses can place in the account.* None of the money placed in an irrevocable burial fund will be counted in determining the ill spouse's Medi-Cal eligibility.

EXAMPLE

Joe and Gina are married. Joe recently had a stroke and will soon enter a nursing home. Their assets consist of their home, which needs at least $15,000 worth of repairs, and $100,000 in a savings account. Joe applied for Medi-Cal benefits and was told by the Eligibility Worker that he cannot qualify because he and his wife have nearly $20,000 in excess assets.

Joe and Gina can protect the $20,000 in excess cash while enabling Joe to qualify for Medi-Cal benefits by using the cash to purchase exempt assets.

For example, the home needs $15,000 worth of repairs. Joe and Gina could spend $15,000 of the excess cash on home repairs. They could also spend the remaining excess funds on burial plots, and revocable and irrevocable burial funds.

STRATEGY B

PURCHASE AN IRREVOCABLE ANNUITY IN THE NAME OF THE WELL SPOUSE

The well spouse can use excess cash or securities to purchase an irrevocable, single-premium annuity in his or her name only. Purchasing an annuity is an extremely effective asset preservation strategy because it protects liquid assets (e.g., cash) while providing a pension-like income stream for the well spouse. As stated in Chapter 2, under the Medi-Cal regulations, the value of money placed in an irrevocable, single premium, immediate annuity will not be counted in determining Medi-Cal eligibility. Such an annuity is required to make periodic distributions of both interest and principal. If the annuity is purchased in the name of the well spouse, Medi-Cal will allow the well spouse to receive all of these income distributions. (See Chapter 5 discussion on the "name on the instrument rule.")

EXAMPLE

John and Mary are married. John is in a nursing home. Their only asset with any monetary value is Certificates of Deposit worth $100,000. John is ineligible to receive Medi-Cal benefits because the value of the couple's non-exempt assets exceeds the Medi-Cal eligibility limit by approximately $20,000.

However, as an alternative to spending down to the eligibility limit, Mary can use $20,000 of their savings to purchase an irrevocable annuity for herself. The annuity must pay her periodically both interest and principal. As a result, the value of the $20,000 annuity will not be counted toward John's Medi-Cal eligibility. **Therefore, John will be eligible to receive Medi-Cal benefits.**

STRATEGY C

TRANSFER ASSETS OUT OF THE COUPLE'S ESTATE

THE "HALF LOAF" TRANSFER STRATEGY
One effective method of protecting cash is known as the "half loaf" strategy. Under this strategy, the couple transfers **half** of their excess assets (e.g., cash) out of their names. Although transferring cash causes a period of ineligibility, under this strategy, the remaining excess cash is used to pay for nursing home care during the period of ineligibility.

There are three advantages to using the half loaf strategy. First, the cash transfer brings the value of the couple's assets closer the Medi-Cal eligibility limit. This is because the transferred cash is no longer counted as an asset owned by the couple.

Second, the cash transferred out of the couple's names can be protected for future use. Although the cash that was transferred must be held in the name of a trusted family member or friend, that person can later use the funds to pay for items or services that are needed, but not financed by Medi-Cal. In fact, the person holding the funds can spend the money on whatever else is deemed necessary for the couple's general well-being.

Third, the transfer will not prevent the ill spouse from receiving the nursing home care that is needed. Although the cash transfer causes a period of ineligibility, the remaining half of the excess cash can be used to pay for the cost of care during the period of ineligibility.

EXAMPLE

John and Mary are married. John enters into a nursing home and applies for Medi-Cal benefits. Their only asset consists of a $120,000 savings account. Thus, the value of their non-exempt assets exceeds the Medi-Cal eligibility limit by approximately $40,000. If they spend down to the Medi-Cal eligibility limit by paying privately for John's nursing home care at $3,882 a month, he will be eligible for Medi-Cal benefits in ten months.

However, John and Mary can use the "half loaf" transfer strategy. This strategy involves transferring half of the excess cash, and retaining the other half to pay for the cost of nursing home care during the resulting period of ineligibility.

Here's how it works: John and Mary have $40,000 in excess assets. Using the "half loaf" strategy, they give $20,000 to their son, Bill for "safe keeping". The period of ineligibility that results from this gift is five months. The $20,000 John and Mary retain will cover the cost of his nursing home care during this six-month period of ineligibility. Thus, John will be eligible for Medi-Cal benefits in only five months, instead of the ten months that it would have taken if the couple had merely spent down to the eligibility limit.

There is an additional advantage to making this "half loaf" transfer. If John and Mary had merely spent the $40,000 in excess assets on John's care, the money would be gone forever. Instead, transferring only half of the money preserves the other $20,000 for future use by John and Mary. For example, Bill can use the funds to pay for items or services that are needed, but not financed by Medi-Cal. In fact, Bill can use the money on whatever else is deemed necessary for the John and Mary's general well-being.

**Payoff Debts
Credit Cards
Mortgages
Outstanding Bills
Promissory Notes
Taxes**

STRATEGY D

PAY OFF DEBTS (EXCEPT UNPAID MEDICAL BILLS)

Another effective strategy to protect excess cash assets is to pay off current debts. Such debts may include credit card debts, mortgages, outstanding utility bills, promissory notes, and taxes. Paying off such debts will reduce the amount of the excess cash. Paying off debts prior to Medi-Cal eligibility will also enable the well spouse to maximize the income that he or she can retain once the ill spouse begins receiving Medi-Cal benefits. This is because once the ill spouse begins receiving Medi-Cal benefits, the well spouse will only be allowed to retain a limited amount of the household income. Consequently, if debts are paid off prior to Medi-Cal eligibility, once eligibility does occur, the well spouse will not need to divert a large portion of his or her limited income to paying debts.

While spending money to pay debts associated with medical bills is permissible, it is advantageous to repay unpaid medical bills once the ill spouse begins receiving Medi-Cal benefits. The reason for this is explained in later in this book when "Income Rules" are discussed.

CAN CAREGIVERS BE REIMBURSED FOR OUT-OF-POCKET COSTS INCURRED IN CARING FOR AN ILL SPOUSE?

Yes. The couple can reimburse friends or family members for out-of-pocket expenses they may have incurred in providing care to the ill spouse. However, in such situations, Medi-Cal could consider some of these reimbursements as "gifts in disguise" and impose a period of ineligibility. To minimize this possibility, there are a few precautions that can be taken.

1) Have a prior written agreement as to which expenses are expected to be reimbursed.

    There should be a signed, written agreement between the couple and the caregiver regarding reimbursement prior to any expenditures by the caregiver. It should clearly state that such expenditures are expected to be reimbursed. (See Appendix IV for a Promissory Note Agreement).

2) Have a detailed record of the costs and reimbursements.

    In addition to a written agreement prior to making any expenditures, make sure that there is a detailed "paper trail" of the actual expenditures and reimbursements. This requires a written record which lists the item purchased, the amount, and the date of the expenditure. It should also state the amount and date of repayment to the caregiver.

3) Make sure the couple is not reimbursing a family member for general living expenses such as room and board. Medi-Cal will not allow reimbursements to caregivers who are family members if the reimbursements are for general living expenses, such as room and board. Medi-Cal expects that close relatives will spend money for general living expenses for their loved ones without the expectation of compensation. An exception to this expectation would be an expense associated with remodeling of the home to accommodate the ill spouse. Other out-of-pocket expenses for medications, special diets, and medical equipment are not general living expenses and, consequently, a caregiver would ordinarily expect reimbursement.

PROMISSORY NOTE

_____ DATE $_____

The undersigned promises to pay to the order of _____

the total sum of ($_____) on demand with interest in the amount

of _____ (_____%) on said sum annually until said sum

is paid in full.

DATE:_____

_____
(signature)

Example:
Promissory Note

Reimbursing friends and/or family members for caregiving expenses carries a high risk of being characterized by Medi-Cal as a gift in disguise—even with these precautions. An attorney knowledgeable in Medi-Cal law could be extremely helpful is providing you with further guidance on what types of reimbursements would be permissible to Medi-Cal.

STRATEGY E

OBTAIN A COURT ORDER

It may be possible for the couple to obtain a court order that increases the amount of non-exempt assets that the couple is allowed to retain above the standard Medi-Cal eligibility limit for married persons. Under State law, a court can increase the amount of assets that the well spouse is allowed to retain if such an increase is necessary for that spouse to have sufficient income for support and maintenance, as defined by the Medi-Cal regulations. Currently, Medi-Cal has determined that the level of income needed for the support and maintenance of the well spouse is $2,049 per month. (see the chapter discussing "Income Rules for Married Persons").

EXAMPLE

John and Mary, a married couple, have a household income of $2,000 per month. Half of their income, or $1,000 per month, is produced from interest they receive on their Certificates of Deposit which are worth $300,000. They have no other assets.

If John enters a nursing home and needs Medi-Cal benefits, a court of law could increase the Medi-Cal eligibility limit for the couple so that they can retain the $300,000 in CDs. The court would have the power to increase the Medi-Cal eligibility limit in this situation because Mary would need the income produced from the CDs to bring the household income to the level that is necessary for her support and maintenance.

This strategy could involve complex court procedures and a thorough knowledge of the Medi-Cal laws and regulations. Therefore, it is highly recommended that an attorney knowledgeable in Medi-Cal be consulted.

NOTE: PROTECTING SECURITIES SUCH AS STOCKS, BONDS, AND MUTUAL FUNDS

The above-listed strategies also apply to protecting securities such as stocks, bonds, and mutual funds. To protect the value of these assets, merely liquidate them to cash, and then implement any of the strategies listed for protecting cash.

ASSET PROTECTION STRATEGIES
PROTECTION OF RENTAL PROPERTY

There are two basic strategies for protecting rental property:

A. TRANSFER THE RENTAL PROPERTY
B. BORROW ON THE PROPERTY

STRATEGY A
TRANSFER THE RENTAL PROPERTY

The couple can transfer the rental property out of their name as a means of reducing the amount of their excess assets—even though such a transfer is likely to incur a period of ineligibility. As stated in the previous chapter, the duration of the period of ineligibility is based on the value of the asset transferred. Thus, transferring rental property may seem to result in a very long period of ineligibility given the high market value of most rental property in California.

However, as stated in the previous chapter, Medi-Cal does not look at the fair market value of the property transferred. It looks at the **net assessed value** of the property transferred in calculating the period of ineligibility. In addition, six thousand dollars are deducted from the net assessed value, if the property produces an annual rental income that is **at least 6 percent of the net assessed value.** Thus, transferring rental property may, in fact, result in only a short period of ineligibility, if any.

EXAMPLE

John and Mary, a married couple, own their home and a single family residence that they use as a rental. The property's assessed value is $40,000. They currently owe $10,000 on the rental. The annual rental produces at least **6 percent of the net assessed value.** thus, the properties qualifies for the six thousand dollar exemption. John enters a nursing home and applies for Medi-Cal benefits.

If the couple transfers the rental property out of their names this gift would only result in a six month period of ineligibility.

This is how Medi-Cal would do the calculation:

Step One: Calculate the net assessed value:

$40,000
−$10,000 (encumbrance)
$30,000 Net Assessed Value

Step Two: Subtract $6,000 from the net assessed value:

$30,000
− $6,000 (exemption)
$24,000

Step Three: Calculate the period of ineligibility
based on a $24,000 transfer of assets:

$24,000
÷ $3,882 avg. monthly private pay rate
6 months (fractions are not counted)

Thus, as illustrated, it is possible to transfer a rental property while incurring a relatively short period of ineligibility.

STRATEGY B

BORROW ON THE PROPERTY

As previously stated, in determining Medi-Cal eligibility, the State will count the net assessed value of the property. Thus, borrowing on the rental property correspondingly reduces the value of the rental that will be counted in determining the ill spouse's Medi-Cal eligibility.

EXAMPLE

John and Mary, a married couple, own their home and a single family residence that they use as a rental. Its assessed value is only $40,000. They currently owe $10,000 on the rental. The annual rental produces **at least 6 percent of the net assessed value**— thus the property qualifies for the six thousand dollar exemption. John enters a nursing home and applies for Medi-Cal benefits.

John became eligible for Medi-Cal benefits without selling or transferring the rental by borrowing on the property in order to reduce its net assessed value.

This is how it would work:

Step One: Calculate the net assessed value:

$40,000
− $10,000 (encumbrance)
$30,000 Net Assessed Value

Step Two: Subtract $6,000 from the net assessed value:

$30,000
− $6,000 (exemption)
$24,000 Amount counted toward
Medi-Cal eligibility.

Step Three: Borrow on the amount that would be counted toward Medi-Cal eligibility.

In this example, the amount of $24,000 will be counted in determining John's Medi-Cal eligibility. **Consequently, John and Mary can borrow an additional $24,000 on the rental, and none of the rental property's value will be counted toward John's Medi-Cal eligibility.**

As a practical matter, borrowing the amount of the net assessed value of the property should not be difficult since the amount of the loan is often based on a percentage of the actual fair market value of the property. For example, if the actual fair market value of John and Mary's home was $120,000, it should not be difficult for him to obtain an additional $24,000 loan on the rental.

IF A MARRIED COUPLE BORROWS ON THE RENTAL PROPERTY, DOES THE CASH THEY RECEIVE COUNT TOWARD THE ILL SPOUSE'S MEDI-CAL ELIGIBILITY?

Yes, the cash received will count toward the ill spouse's Medi-Cal eligibility. However, the cash received from the loan can be protected by using any of the above stated strategies for protecting cash assets.

ASSET PROTECTION STRATEGIES
PROTECTION OF RETIREMENT ACCOUNTS

A HUSBAND AND WIFE EACH HAVE AN INDIVIDUAL RETIREMENT ACCOUNT. IS THERE ANY WAY THEY CAN PROTECT THEIR RETIREMENT ACCOUNTS?
Receive Periodic Distributions

STRATEGY

RECEIVE PERIODIC DISTRIBUTIONS

The ill spouse should receive periodic distributions from his or her retirement account. Under the Medi-Cal regulations, the value of cash and securities held in retirement accounts, such as IRAs and 401(K)s, is not counted if the account is owned by the well spouse. If the retirement account is owned by the ill spouse, the account will also be exempt as long as the person applying for Medi-Cal benefits is periodically receiving a distribution of both interest and principal from the account.

Therefore, in protecting the value of the ill spouse's retirement account, it is critical to that he or she begins receiving a periodic distribution from this account before applying Medi-Cal benefits. Even a small periodic distribution of both interest and principal is sufficient to make the entire value of this account exempt. Again, retirement accounts of the well spouse are automatically exempt—he or she need not receive a distribution.

EXAMPLE

John and Mary Smith each have IRAs. John has $50,000 in his IRA. Mary has $40,000 in her IRA. Neither spouse receives a distribution.

If John enters a nursing home and needs Medi-Cal benefits, the value of his IRA can be protected if John begins receiving periodic distributions of both interest and principal from his IRA.

Under the Medi-Cal regulations, once John begins receiving these distributions, the principal value of his IRA will be exempt.

Since Mary is the well spouse, the value of her IRA is automatically exempt.

ASSET PROTECTION STRATEGIES

PROTECTION OF WHOLE LIFE INSURANCE

A HUSBAND AND WIFE EACH HAVE LIFE INSURANCE POLICIES THAT HAVE ACCUMULATED CASH VALUE. HOW CAN THIS CASH BE PROTECTED?
Remove Cash Value From The Policy.

STRATEGY

REMOVE CASH VALUE FROM THE POLICY

Under the Medi-Cal regulations, if the face value of each spouse's Whole Life Insurance policies exceeds $1,500, the cash surrender value of the policy is counted toward the $83,960 Medi-Cal eligibility limit. Therefore, if the face value of either spouse's life insurance exceeds the $1,500 limit, he or she can remove the cash from the policy, and thus reduce the cash surrender value. Once the couple has the cash, they can employ any of the above strategies for protecting cash assets.

EXAMPLE

John and Mary are married. John recently entered into a nursing home and applied for Medi-Cal benefits. John and Mary each have life insurance policies. John's life insurance policy has a face value of $20,000 and a cash surrender value of $10,000. Mary life insurance policy has a face value of $1,000 and a cash surrender value of $500. Since the face value of John's life insurance exceeds the $1,500 limit, the cash surrender value of his policy will be counted toward the $83,960 Medi-Cal eligibility limit. The face value of Mary's life insurance policy is within the $1,500 limit. Thus, its cash surrender value will not be counted toward the Medi-Cal eligibility limit.

John can protect the cash value of his life insurance by removing the $10,000 from the policy and thus reduce its cash surrender value to zero.

Once the couple have the $10,000 cash in their possession, they could then employ any of the asset protection strategies stated above for protecting cash. For example, the couple could use the $10,000 to purchase a burial plots and to establish revocable and irrevocable burial funds.

ARE MY WIFE AND I LIMITED TO USING ONLY ONE ASSET PROTECTION STRATEGY?

Absolutely not. Either one strategy, or a combination of the strategies listed, could be very effective in protecting your assets. (Please read the Appendix containing a sample Medi-Cal Plan for an example of using a combination of asset protection strategies)

SHOULD A MARRIED COUPLE SPEND ANY OF THEIR MONEY ON AN ILL SPOUSE'S NURSING HOME CARE BEFORE APPLYING FOR MEDI-CAL BENEFITS?

Yes, if possible. Having the ill spouse enter the nursing home as a "private pay patient" for three to six months before converting to Medi-Cal could have a very practical benefit. Experience has indicated that it is easier to gain admission into a quality nursing home facility if your ill spouse enters as a private pay patient. The likely reason for the nursing home facility's reluctance to admit Medi-Cal patients is that Medi-Cal reimburses the nursing home at a lower rate than the rate paid by private pay patients. Therefore, it may be prudent for the couple to plan to spend approximately $12,000 to $18,000 on the cost of the ill spouse's care before applying for Medi-Cal benefits. This amount should pay for three to six months of nursing home care.

After the ill spouse is admitted into the nursing home, and pays privately for three to six months, then he or she can convert to Medi-Cal. It is important to note that Medi-Cal patients are intermingled with private pay patients; they are not placed in a separate section of the nursing home. Under the law, Medi-Cal patients must receive the same quality of care as private pay patients.

Section 1: SUMMARY

The potential danger of the "spend down" option is that the well spouse may not be left with sufficient assets to meet his or her financial, personal, and health care needs. The following are the various asset protection strategies that serve as alternatives to the traditional "spend down" option.

STRATEGIES FOR PROTECTING CASH AND/OR SECURITIES:
a. Purchase Exempt Assets.
b. Purchase an Irrevocable Annuity.
c. Transfer Cash and/or Securities.
d. Pay off Debts (Except Medical Bills).

STRATEGIES FOR PROTECTING RENTAL PROPERTY:
a. Transfer the rental property.
b. Borrow on the rental property and use strategies for protecting cash.

STRATEGY FOR PROTECTING RETIREMENT ACCOUNTS:
Receive periodic distributions from the retirement accounts.

STRATEGY FOR PROTECTING CASH VALUE
FROM LIFE INSURANCE:
Remove the cash value from the life insurance and use strategies for protecting cash.

The couple is not limited to using one of these asset protection strategies. One or more of these strategies can be used consecutively or concurrently.

Although the asset protection strategies can effectively render the ill spouse Medi-Cal eligible, your loved one is likely to have greater access to a quality nursing facility if he or she can first enter as a private pay patient. Therefore, if possible, the couple should plan to pay for the ill spouse's care for approximately three to six months before applying for Medi-Cal benefits.

SECTION II

ASSET PROTECTION STRATEGIES FOR SINGLE PERSONS

WHAT HAPPENS IF MY LOVED ONE HAS ASSETS WHICH EXCEED THE MEDI-CAL ELIGIBILITY LIMIT?

If an ill person has assets in excess of the Medi-Cal eligibility limit, he or she is ineligible to receive Medi-Cal benefits. In this situation, the State prefers for the ill person to pay the nursing home for the cost of his or her care until the ill person has spent down to the $2,000 Medi-Cal eligibility limit.

WHAT IS THE DANGER OF SPENDING DOWN TO THE ELIGIBILITY LIMIT?

The potential danger of the "spend down" option is that the ill person may not be left with sufficient assets to meet his or her financial, personal, and health care needs. In addition, since Medi-Cal does not pay every health care cost, there may be medical procedures or equipment that the ill person needs that are not covered by Medi-Cal. If the ill person has spent down to the Medi-Cal eligibility limit, then he or she may not have sufficient assets to pay for these needed procedures or equipment.

ARE THERE ANY ALTERNATIVES TO SPENDING DOWN TO THE MEDI-CAL ELIGIBILITY LIMIT?

There are various asset protection strategies that serve as alternatives to the traditional "spend down" option. The following are some proven strategies that can effectively protect assets for the ill person, while enabling him or her to become Medi-Cal eligible. Either one strategy, or a combination of the strategies listed, may be useful. However, the appropriateness of each asset protection strategy depends on the type and nature of the asset to be protected. For example, strategies to protect cash are different from strategies to protect real estate.

ASSET PROTECTION STRATEGIES
PROTECTION OF CASH/SECURITIES

There are five basic strategies that can be used to protect the ill person's excess cash.

A. **CONVERT CASH INTO EXEMPT ASSETS.**

B. **PURCHASE AN IRREVOCABLE ANNUITY IN THE NAME OF THE ILL PERSON.**

C. **TRANSFER ASSETS OUT OF THE ILL PERSON'S ESTATE.**

D. **PAY OFF DEBTS (EXCEPT UNPAID MEDICAL BILLS).**

STRATEGY A

CONVERT CASH INTO EXEMPT ASSETS

The ill person can convert the excess cash into exempt assets. This is accomplished by using cash assets to purchase exempt assets. For example, if the non-exempt assets exceed the Medi-Cal eligibility limit but the ill person has a mortgage, the excess cash can be used to pay off the mortgage. The same principle applies to home repairs, remodeling the home, paying attorney's fees, purchasing personal jewelry and household items, purchasing burial plots, and establishing burial funds.

In addition, the ill person can purchase revocable and irrevocable burial funds. A revocable burial fund is a separate trust fund or savings account in which the funds are used to pay for burial expenses. One can place funds in a revocable burial fund and later terminate the fund if he or she desires. Monies placed in a revocable burial fund will not be counted in determining the ill person's Medi-Cal eligibility if the value of the fund does not exceed $1,500.

The ill person can also purchase an irrevocable burial fund. Irrevocable burial funds are trust funds that are used for burial expenses. However, once the person places the funds in the account, he or she cannot later terminate the account. **Unlike revocable burial funds, there is no limit on the amount the person can place in the account.** None of the money placed in an irrevocable burial fund will be counted in determining the ill person's Medi-Cal eligibility.

EXAMPLE

Joe recently had a stroke and will soon enter a nursing home. His assets consist of his home, which needs at least $10,000 worth of repairs, and $20,000 in a savings account. Joe applied for Medi-Cal benefits and was told by the Eligibility Worker that he cannot qualify because he has nearly $20,000 in excess assets.

Joe can protect the $20,000 in excess cash while qualifying for Medi-Cal benefits by using the excess cash to purchase exempt assets.

In this example, the home needs $15,000 worth of repairs. Joe could spend $15,000 of the excess cash on home repairs. He could spend the remaining excess funds on a burial plot, and revocable and irrevocable burial funds.

STRATEGY B

PURCHASE AN IRREVOCABLE ANNUITY IN THE NAME OF THE ILL PERSON

The ill person can use excess cash or securities to purchase an irrevocable, single-premium annuity in his or her name. Purchasing an annuity is an extremely effective asset preservation strategy because it protects liquid assets (e.g., cash) while providing a pension-like income stream for the ill person.

As stated in Chapter 2, under the Medi-Cal regulations, the value of money placed in an irrevocable, single premium, immediate annuity will not be counted in determining Medi-Cal eligibility. Such an annuity is required to make periodic distributions of both interest and principal.

EXAMPLE

John, a widower, is in a nursing home. John's only assets with any monetary value are Certificates of Deposit worth $30,000. John is ineligible to receive Medi-Cal benefits because the value of his non-exempt assets exceeds the Medi-Cal eligibility limit by approximately $28,000.

However, as an alternative to spending down to the eligibility limit, John can use $28,000 of his savings to purchase an irrevocable annuity for himself. Consequently, the value of the $28,000 annuity will not be counted toward John's Medi-Cal eligibility. Thus, **John will be eligible to receive Medi-Cal benefits.**

STRATEGY C

TRANSFER ASSETS OUT OF THE ILL PERSON'S ESTATE

One effective method of protecting cash is known as the "half loaf" strategy. Under this strategy, the ill person transfers half of his or her excess cash. Although transferring cash causes a period of ineligibility, under this strategy, the remaining excess cash is used to pay for nursing home care during the period of ineligibility.

There are three advantages to using the "half loaf" strategy. First, the cash transfer brings the value of the ill person's assets closer the Medi-Cal eligibility limit. This is because the transferred cash is no longer counted as an asset owned by the ill person.

Second, the cash transferred out of the ill person's name will be available for future use. Although the cash that was transferred must be held in the name of a trusted family member or friend, that person can later use the funds to pay for items or services that are needed, but not financed by Medi-Cal. In fact, the person holding the funds can spend the money on whatever else is deemed necessary for the ill person's general well-being.

Third, the transfer will not prevent the ill person from receiving the nursing home care that they need. Although the cash transfer causes a period of ineligibility, the remaining half of the excess cash can be used to pay for the cost of care during the period of ineligibility.

EXAMPLE

John, a widower, enters into a nursing home. His only asset is a savings account with a balance of $40,000. Thus, the value of his non-exempt assets exceeds the Medi-Cal eligibility limit by $38,000. If he spends down to the Medi-Cal eligibility limit by paying privately for nursing home care at $3,800 a month, he will be eligible for Medi-Cal benefits in approximately ten months, and his savings will be exhausted.

However, if John uses the "half loaf" transfer strategy, he will become eligible for Medi-Cal benefits in only 5 months, while protecting some of the cash for his personal needs.

Here's how it works:

John has $40,000 in savings. He gives $20,000 to his son, Bill, for "safe keeping." The period of ineligibility that results from this gift is 5 months. The $20,000 that John retains will cover the cost of his nursing home care during the five-month period of ineligibility.

Thus, John will be eligible for Medi-Cal in only five months, instead of the ten months that it would have taken if he had merely spent down to the $2,000 eligibility limit. Moreover, $20,000 has been preserved since it is in Bill's name. Bill can use the $20,000 to pay for items or services that his father might need, but are not financed by Medi-Cal. In fact, Bill can use the funds to pay for whatever else is deemed necessary for John's care and general well-being.

STRATEGY D

PAY OFF DEBTS (EXCEPT UNPAID MEDICAL BILLS)

Payoff Debts
Credit Cards
Mortgages
Outstanding Bills
Promissory Notes
Taxes

Another effective strategy to protect excess cash assets is to pay off current debts. Such debts may include credit card debts, mortgages, outstanding utility bills, promissory notes, and taxes. Paying off such debts will reduce the amount of the excess cash. Paying off debts prior to Medi-Cal eligibility will also enable the ill person to maximize the income that he or she can retain once the ill person begins receiving Medi-Cal benefits. This is because, once the ill person begins receiving Medi-Cal benefits, the ill person will only be allowed to retain $35.00 per month of income. Consequently, once eligibility does occur, the ill person will not have the opportunity to pay debts.

While spending money to pay debts associated with medical bills is permissible, it is advantageous to repay unpaid medical bills once the ill person begins receiving Medi-Cal benefits. The reason for this is explained in Chapter 5: MEDI-CAL INCOME RULES.

CAN CAREGIVERS BE REIMBURSED FOR OUT-OF-POCKET COSTS INCURRED IN CARING FOR THE ILL PERSON?

Yes. The ill person can reimburse friends or family members for out-of-pocket expenses they may have incurred in providing care to the ill person. However, in such situations, Medi-Cal could consider some of these reimbursements as "gifts in disguise" and impose a period of ineligibility. To minimize this possibility, there are a few precautions that can be taken:

1) Have a prior written agreement as to which expenses are expected to be reimbursed.

   There should be a signed, written agreement between the ill person and the caregiver regarding reimbursement prior to any expenditures by the caregiver. It should clearly state that such expenditures are expected to be reimbursed. (See the Appendix IV for a Promissory Note Agreement).

2) Have a detailed record of the costs and reimbursements.

   In addition to a written agreement prior to making any expenditures, make sure that there is a detailed "paper trail" of the actual expenditures

Example:
Promissory Note

PROMISSORY NOTE

_____ DATE $_____

The undersigned promises to pay to the order of _____
the total sum of ($_____) on demand with interest in the amount
of _____ (_____%) on said sum annually until said sum
is paid in full.

                              DATE:_____

                              _____
                              (signature)

and reimbursements. This requires a written record which lists the item purchased, the amount and the date of the expenditure. It should also state the amount and date of repayment to the caregiver.

3) Make sure the ill person is not reimbursing a family member for general living expenses such as room and board.

Medi-Cal will not allow reimbursements to caregivers who are family members if the reimbursements are for general living expenses such as room and board. Medi-Cal expects close relatives to spend money for general living expenses for their loved ones without the expectation of compensation. An exception to this expectation would be an expense associated with remodeling of the home to accommodate the ill person. Other out-of-pocket expenses for medications, special diets, and medical equipment are not general living expenses. Therefore, a caregiver would ordinarily expect reimbursement.

Reimbursing friends and/or family members for caregiving expenses carries a high risk of being characterized by Medi-Cal as a gift in disguise—even with these precautions. An attorney knowledgeable in Medi-Cal law could be extremely helpful is providing you with further guidance on what types of reimbursements would be permissible to Medi-Cal.

HOW CAN MY LOVED ONE PROTECT HIS OR HER MUTUAL FUNDS, CERTIFICATES OF DEPOSIT, STOCKS AND OTHER SECURITIES?

The above listed strategies also apply to protecting securities such as stocks, bonds, and mutual funds. To protect the value of these assets, merely liquidate them to cash, and then implement any of the strategies listed for protecting cash.

ASSET PROTECTION STRATEGIES
PROTECTION OF RENTAL PROPERTY

There are two basic strategies that can be used to protect rental property:

A. TRANSFER THE RENTAL PROPERTY
B. BORROW ON THE PROPERTY

STRATEGY A
TRANSFER THE RENTAL PROPERTY

The ill person can transfer the rental property out of his or her name as a means of reducing the amount of their excess assets. This is a particularly vital strategy for single persons who own rental property. Since the Medi-Cal eligibility limit for single persons is only $2,000, the ill person is almost guaranteed to be determined ineligible for Medi-Cal benefits if he or she owns any rental property. In such cases, Medi-Cal would typically advise the ill person to sell the rental, and spend down to the Medi-Cal eligibility limit—thus, the rental could be lost without this asset protection strategy.

Although transferring the rental is likely to produce a period of ineligibility, the duration of the period may be relatively short. As stated in the previous chapter, the duration of the period of ineligibility is based on the value of the asset transferred.

However, as stated in the previous chapter, Medi-Cal does not look at the fair market value of the property transferred; it looks at the **net assessed value** of the property transferred in calculating the period of ineligibility. In addition, six thousand dollars are deducted from the net assessed value, if the property produces an annual rental income that is **at least 6 percent of the net assessed value.** Thus, transferring rental property may, in fact, result in only a short period of ineligibility.

EXAMPLE

John owns his home. He also owns a single family home that he uses as a rental. Although its market value is $120,000, its assessed value is only $40,000. He currently owes $10,000 on the rental. The annual rental produces **at least 6 percent of the net assessed value,** –thus qualifying the property for the six thousand dollar exemption. Recently, John entered a nursing home and applied for Medi-Cal benefits.

If John transfers the rental property out of his name, he will only incur a six month period of ineligibility.

This is how Medi-Cal would do the calculation:

Step One: Determine the net assessed value of the property:

$40,000
– $10,000 (encumbrance)
$30,000 Net Assessed Value

Step Two: Subtract the $6,000 Exemption from the net assessed value:

$30,000
– $6,000 (exemption)
$24,000 Value of Rental

Step Three: Calculate the period of ineligibility based on the value of the rental transferred:

$24,000
÷ $3,882 avg. monthly private pay rate
6 months (fractions are not counted)

Thus, as illustrated, it is possible to transfer a rental property while incurring a relatively short period of ineligibility.

STRATEGY B

BORROW ON THE PROPERTY

As previously stated, the State will count the net assessed value of the rental property (minus the $6,000 exclusion) in determining Medi-Cal eligibility. Therefore another effective strategy is for the ill person to borrow on the rental property and thus reduce its net assessed value.

EXAMPLE

John, a widower, owns his home. His only other asset is a single family residence that he uses as a rental. The rental's net assessed value is $36,000. Because the rental produces at least 6 percent of the net assessed value in annual income, the property qualifies for the $6,000 deduction. Thus, the countable value of the rental is $30,000.

John can become eligible for Medi-Cal benefits without selling or transferring the rental if he borrows on the rental and uses the asset protection strategies for protecting cash.

Consequently, John can borrow $30,000 on the rental, and none of the rental's value will be counted toward John's Medi-Cal eligibility.

As a practical matter, borrowing the amount of the net assessed value of the property should not be difficult since the amount of the loan is often based on a percentage of the actual fair market value of the property. For example, if the actual fair market value of John's home was $120,000, it should be difficult for him to obtain an additional $30,000 loan on the rental property.

IF THE ILL PERSON BORROWS ON THE RENTAL PROPERTY, DOES THE CASH RECEIVED COUNT TOWARD HIS OR HER MEDI-CAL ELIGIBILITY?

Yes, the cash received will count toward the ill person's Medi-Cal eligibility. However, the cash received from the loan can be protected by using any of the above stated strategies for protecting cash assets.

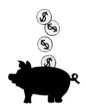

ASSET PROTECTION STRATEGIES
PROTECTION OF RETIREMENT ACCOUNTS

MY LOVED ONE HAS AN INDIVIDUAL RETIREMENT ACCOUNT. IS THERE ANY WAY TO PROTECT THIS ASSET?
A. Receive Periodic Distributions

STRATEGY

RECEIVE PERIODIC DISTRIBUTIONS

Your loved one should receive periodic distributions from his or her retirement account. Under the Medi-Cal regulations, the retirement account will be exempt as long as the owner of the account is periodically receiving a distribution of both interest and principal. Even a small periodic distribution of both interest and principal is sufficient to make the entire value of this account exempt.

EXAMPLE

John, a widower, has an IRA worth $30,000. He does not receive a distribution from the account. If John enters a nursing home and needs Medi-Cal, the value of John's IRAs can be protected if he elects to receive periodic distributions of both interest and principal from his IRA. Once he begins receiving these distributions, the principal value of his IRA will be exempt.

ASSET PROTECTION STRATEGIES
PROTECTION OF WHOLE LIFE INSURANCE

MY LOVED ONE HAS LIFE INSURANCE POLICIES THAT HAVE ACCUMULATED CASH VALUE. HOW CAN THIS CASH BE PROTECTED?

STRATEGY

REMOVE CASH VALUE FROM THE POLICY

Under the Medi-Cal regulations, if the face value of an ill person's Whole Life Insurance policies exceeds $1,500, the cash surrender value of the policies is counted toward the $2,000 Medi-Cal eligibility limit. Therefore, if the face value of the ill person's life insurance policy exceeds the $1,500 limit, he or she can remove the cash from the policy, and thus reduce its cash surrender value. Once your loved one has the cash, he or she can employ any of the above strategies for protecting cash assets.

EXAMPLE

John recently entered into a nursing home and applied for Medi-Cal benefits. John's life insurance policy has a face value of $20,000, and a cash surrender value of $10,000. Since the face value of John's life insurance exceeds the $1,500 limit, the cash surrender value of his policy will be counted toward the $2,000 Medi-Cal eligibility limit.

John can protect the cash value of his life insurance by removing the $10,000 from the policy, thereby reducing the cash surrender value to zero.

John could then protect the $10,000 in cash by using any of the asset protection strategies previously described for protecting cash. For example, John could use the $10,000 to purchase a burial plot, establish revocable and irrevocable burial funds, and pay off debts.

IS MY LOVED ONE LIMITED TO USING ONLY ONE ASSET PROTECTION STRATEGY?

Absolutely not. Either one strategy, or a combination of the strategies listed, could be very effective in protecting the assets of your loved one. (Please see the Appendix I for Medi-Cal Plans for examples of using a combination of asset protection strategies).

SHOULD MY LOVED ONE SPEND ANY OF HIS OR HER MONEY ON NURSING HOME CARE BEFORE APPLYING FOR MEDI-CAL BENEFITS?

Yes, if possible. Having the ill person enter the nursing home as a "private pay patient" for three to six months before converting to Medi-Cal could have a very practical benefit. Experience has indicated that it is easier to gain admission into a quality nursing home facility if your loved one enters as a private pay patient. The likely reason for the nursing home facility's reluctance to admit Medi-Cal patients is that Medi-Cal reimburses the nursing home at a lower rate than the rate paid by private pay patients. Therefore, if possible, the ill person should plan to spend approximately $12,000 to $18,000 on the cost of his or her care before applying for Medi-Cal benefits. This amount should pay for three to six months of nursing home care.

After the ill person is admitted into the nursing home, and pays privately for three to six months, then he or she can convert to Medi-Cal. It is important to note that Medi-Cal patients are intermingled with private pay patients; they are not placed in a separate section of the nursing home. Under the law, Medi-Cal patients must receive the same quality of care as private pay patients.

Section II: SUMMARY

The potential danger of the "spend down" option is that the ill person may not be left with sufficient assets to meet his or her financial, personal, and health care needs. The following are the various asset protection strategies that serve as alternatives to the traditional "spend down" option.

STRATEGIES FOR PROTECTING CASH AND/OR SECURITIES :
   a. Purchase Exempt Assets.
   b. Purchase an Irrevocable Annuity.
   c. Transfer Cash and/or Securities.
   d. Pay off Debts (Except Medical Bills).

STRATEGIES FOR PROTECTING RENTAL PROPERTY:
   a. Transfer the rental property.
   b. Borrow on the rental property and use strategies for protecting cash.

STRATEGY FOR PROTECTING RETIREMENT ACCOUNTS:

Receive periodic distributions from the retirement accounts.

STRATEGY FOR PROTECTING CASH VALUE FROM LIFE INSURANCE:

Remove the cash value from the life insurance and use strategies for protecting cash.

Your loved one is not limited to using one of these asset protection strategies. One or more of these strategies can be used consecutively or concurrently.

Although the asset protection strategies can effectively render your loved Medi-Cal eligible, your loved one is likely to have greater access to a quality nursing facility if he or she can first enter as a private pay patient. Therefore, if possible, the ill person should plan to pay for their care for approximately three to six months before applying for Medi-Cal benefits.

CHAPTER 4

PROTECTING THE HOME FROM MEDI-CAL ESTATE CLAIMS

This chapter covers the following topics:

General rules regarding Medi-Cal Estate Claims

Strategies for Protecting the Home from a Medi-Cal Estate Claim

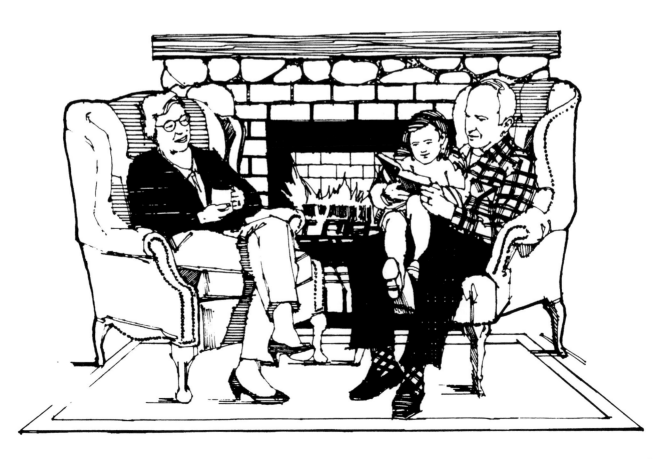

SECTION I

PROTECTING THE HOME FROM MEDI-CAL ESTATE CLAIMS
For Married Persons

IF THE ILL SPOUSE RECEIVES MEDI-CAL BENEFITS AND LATER DIES, CAN THE STATE TAKE THE COUPLE'S HOME?

Under the Medi-Cal regulations, the State can make a claim on a Medi-Cal recipient's estate in order to recover the cost of the Medi-Cal benefits provided. Upon the death of the Medi-Cal recipient, the Department of Health Services is entitled to collect the lesser of the following:

1) the cost of the Medi-Cal benefits provided, or

2) the value of the ill spouse's estate at the time of death. In either case, **the State cannot make a claim on the estate until the surviving spouse has died.**

Although the home is an "exempt" asset for the purposes of Medi-Cal eligibility, its value will be subject to an estate claim. The practical consequence of this rule is that the home must usually be sold upon the death of the surviving spouse so that the estate will have enough money to pay the Medi-Cal estate claim. The State, however, will not demand the home itself.

EXAMPLE

John and Mary Smith owned their home as "joint tenants". John was in a nursing home and receiving Medi-Cal benefits when he died. Their home was worth $100,000. The cost of John's care to the State was $75,000.

The amount of the estate claim is derived as follows:

Step One: Determine the cost to the State of the Medi-Cal benefits provided.

In this example, the cost to the State for John's care was $75,000.

Step Two: Determine the value of the Medi-Cal recipient's estate at the time of death.

In this example, John owned the home jointly with Mary, his wife. Since the home was worth $100,000 when he died, the value of his share was worth $50,000.

Step Three: Compare the two amounts. The lesser number is the amount of the estate claim.

In the example, the cost of the Medi-Cal benefits was $75,000. The value of John's estate was $50,000.

Therefore, **the amount of the estate claim is $50,000.**

As a final note, **the State will not make a $50,000 estate claim until the death of Mary, his surviving spouse.** When the State makes an estate claim, it will not demand the home. Generally, the State will require the sale of the home to satisfy the $50,000 estate claim, unless there is enough money in the estate to satisfy the claim.

CAN MEDI-CAL MAKE AN ESTATE CLAIM WHEN THE COUPLE HAVE A LIVING TRUST WITH NAMED BENEFICIARIES OF THE TRUST PROPERTY?

Yes. Upon the death of the Medi-Cal recipient, the State will make a claim upon the estate. The fact that there is a living trust with named beneficiaries of the trust property is irrelevant to the State. As a creditor of the deceased person, the State is entitled to collect against the property in the Medi-Cal recipient's trust–after the death of the second spouse. Therefore, if there is property in the trust at the time of the Medi-Cal recipient's death, his or her share of the trust property must be used to satisfy the estate claim.after the death of the second spouse. After the estate claim is paid, then any remaining property can be distributed to the named beneficiaries in accordance with the terms written in the trust.

EXAMPLE

Joe Smith, 87, was in a nursing home and received Medi-Cal benefits. He and his wife, Sarah, had a living trust which named their two adult children, Joseph Jr. and Samantha, as beneficiaries of the trust property. The only property in the trust was their home, valued at $100,000. Upon Joe's death, the State imposed a $50,000 Medi-Cal estate claim to be collected after Sarah's death.

Upon Sarah's death, the State is entitled to collect $50,000 from the living trust. The fact that their children are the sole beneficiaries to the living trust is irrelevant. Since the State is a creditor, it is entitled to collect the amount owned from the living trust. Since the only property in the living trust was the home, it would have to be sold, and the estate claim would be satisfied with $50,000 from the proceeds of the sale. The remaining $50,000 would be distributed to Joe and Sarah's two children as the beneficiaries of their trust.

WHAT IF THE TRUST PROPERTY WAS DISTRIBUTED TO THE BENEFICIARIES BEFORE THE STATE COULD COLLECT THE ESTATE CLAIM? CAN THE STATE COLLECT AGAINST THE BENEFICIARIES?

Yes. If the property in the trust is distributed to the beneficiaries prior to satisfying the estate claim, the beneficiaries will be responsible for paying the estate claim, up to the amount of the value of the property that they received from the trust.

EXAMPLE

Joseph Smith, 87, was in a nursing home and received Medi-Cal benefits. He and his wife, Sarah, had a living trust which named their two adult children, Joseph Jr. and Samantha, as beneficiaries of the trust property. The only property in the trust was their home, valued at $100,000. Upon Joe's death, the State imposed a $50,000 Medi-Cal estate claim to be collected upon the death of his wife, Sarah.

Upon Sarah's death, the trust distributed the home to their beneficiaries: Joseph Jr. and Samantha.

The State is entitled to collect $50,000 from Joseph Jr. and Samantha. It is up to Joseph Jr. and Samantha as to how they will pay the estate claim. They could sell or borrow on the home they inherited, or they could pay the estate claim out of their own personal funds. The point is that since Joseph's children received the property before the estate claim was paid, the State will hold them responsible for paying the estate claim, up to the value of the property they received.

AFTER THE DEATH OF THE SECOND SPOUSE, ARE THERE ANY CIRCUMSTANCES IN WHICH THE STATE CANNOT MAKE AN ESTATE CLAIM?

Yes. There are two circumstances in which the State cannot make an estate claim. The first is when the heir or beneficiary of the estate is a minor child of the deceased Medi-Cal recipient. A minor is considered a person under the age of twenty-one. The other circumstance is when the heir or beneficiary is an adult child of the deceased Medi-Cal recipient who is both permanently and totally disabled.

WHEN IS A PERSON PERMANENTLY AND TOTALLY DISABLED FOR THE PURPOSE OF BEING EXEMPTED FROM AN ESTATE CLAIM?

The Medi-Cal regulations do not specifically define "permanently and totally disabled." However, if the adult child whose sole source of income is either SSI (Supplemental Security Income) or Social Security Disability, he or she is likely to qualify for the estate claim exemption.

CAN THE STATE PLACE A LIEN ON THE HOME PRIOR TO THE DEATH OF THE WELL SPOUSE?

If the well spouse continues to live in the home, the State cannot place a lien on the home. Upon the death of the surviving spouse, the State may place a lien on the home for the amount of the estate claim.

CAN LIFE INSURANCE AND ANNUITIES BE PROTECTED FROM A MEDI-CAL ESTATE CLAIM?

Under current practice, Medi-Cal will not make an estate claim on the proceeds of life insurance or annuities.

IS THERE ANY WAY THE COUPLE CAN PROTECT THE VALUE OF THE HOME FROM A MEDI-CAL ESTATE CLAIM?

Yes. There are strategies that the couple can undertake that can avoid, or at least minimize, the effect of a Medi-Cal estate claim. The following strategies may be used to protect the home.

STRATEGY A

TRANSFER THE ILL SPOUSE'S INTEREST IN THE HOME TO THE WELL SPOUSE.

As stated previously, under the Medi-Cal regulations, the amount of the estate claim will be the lesser of the following:

1) the cost of the Medi-Cal benefits provided, or

2) the value of the ill spouse's estate at the time of death.

Therefore, the ill spouse can transfer his or her share in the home to the well spouse. Consequently, at the time of the ill spouse's death, the value of the ill spouse's estate will be zero. Thus, the value of the home will be protected from a Medi-Cal estate claim.

EXAMPLE

John and Mary Smith owned their home as "joint tenants". At the time of John's death, the home was worth $100,000. However, before John's death, he transferred his entire share of the home to Mary. When John died, he was in a nursing home and receiving Medi-Cal benefits. **The cost of John's care to the State was $100,000.**

The amount of the estate claim is zero.

The maximum amount that the State can collect is the value of the assets owned by John at the time of his death or the cost of the Medi-Cal benefits provided—whichever is less. Since the value of John's estate at the time of death was zero, this lower amount must be the amount of the estate claim. Although, the State paid $100,000 for the cost of his care, the State cannot recover the cost from Mary or her heirs.

DOESN'T THIS TRANSFER OF THE HOME CAUSE A PERIOD OF INELIGIBILITY FOR THE ILL SPOUSE?

No. Under the Medi-Cal regulations, gifts of assets between spouses **do not result** in a period of ineligibility.

WHAT CAN I DO IF MY WIFE WHO IS IN A NURSING HOME LACKS SUFFICIENT MENTAL CAPACITY TRANSFER HER INTEREST IN THE HOME?

An ill spouse cannot legally transfer the home if she lacks sufficient mental capacity to sign a deed. If the ill spouse lacks sufficient capacity to sign a deed, there are several possible alternatives:

1) The Living Trust

   Most married persons own their home as community property. Thus, transferring an interest in the home to her spouse will require the ill spouse to have sufficient mental capacity to sign a deed. Alternatively, someone else will need to have sufficient legal authority to sign on the ill spouse's behalf.

   If the couple has a living trust, the trust may give the trustee or successor trustee the necessary legal authority to transfer the interest in the home. The attorney who drafted the trust should be consulted.

2) Durable Power of Attorney for Financial Management

   If the ill spouse has signed a Durable Power of Attorney for Financial Management, this document may provide the agent with the necessary legal authority to transfer the interest in the home. However, the attorney who drafted the Durable Power of Attorney for Financial Management should be consulted. (See Forms and Appendix IV)

3) Conservatorship

   If the ill spouse is under a conservatorship, the appointed conservator may have the legal authority to transfer the ill spouse's interest in the home. However, such transfers usually require the conservator to obtain special permission from the court having jurisdiction over the conservatorship. The attorney representing the conservator or the conservatee should be consulted.

4) Court Order to Transfer Community Property Interest to Spouse with Capacity.

   If the home is owned as community property, there is a special order that the couple can obtain from the county's Superior Court which allows the transfer of an interest in community property from an incapacitated spouse to a competent spouse. Thus, this court order could allow the incapacitated spouse to transfer her interest in the home to her spouse. Obtaining such a court order generally requires the expertise of a lawyer knowledgeable in such matters. Attorneys who practice elder law, estate planning, or family law should be consulted.

STRATEGY B

THE COUPLE TRANSFERS THEIR HOME AND RETAINS A LIFE ESTATE.

Transferring the home and retaining a life estate will at least partially protect the value of the home from the estate claim. A life estate is an interest in real estate that allows the holders of the life estate, known a the life tenants, the right to occupy the property for the remainder of their lives. Upon the death of the life tenants, the life estate is terminated and the actual owner of the property then receives the right to occupy the property.

Transferring the home and retaining a life estate will at least partially protect the value of the home from the estate claim because only the value of the Medi-Cal recipient's interest in the life estate is subject to the estate claim. Moreover, the State is unlikely to enforce an estate against the Medi-Cal recipient's interest in a life estate because of the difficulty in placing an actual value on a life estate.

Nevertheless, the State retains a right to collect against the Medi-Cal recipient's share in the life estate, for this reason, this strategy does not fully protect the value of the home as effectively as an complete transfer of the home to the well spouse.†

†Note: As in the previous strategy, the ill spouse must also have sufficient mental capacity to transfer his or her interest in the home, even if he or she is retaining a life estate.. Also, if this strategy is used, it is suggested that the recipients of the home sign an affidavit stating that the ill spouse can return home whenever he or she wishes and it is medically feasible to do so. (See Affidavit in the Appendix).

STRATEGY C

DO NOTHING AND APPLY FOR A HARDSHIP WAIVER UPON THE DEATH OF THE SURVIVING SPOUSE.

If the ill spouse's interest in the home remains in her name at the time of death, the value of her share in the property would be subject to an estate claim. However, upon the death of the surviving spouse, the recipient of home can apply to the State for a "hardship waiver". This waiver asks the State of California to waive its right to make an estate claim because it would result in significant financial hardship to the heirs. Other factors such as delaying the institutionalization of the ill spouse because of care provided by the heirs will also be considered. The State would then have the option of collecting against the estate or waiving its right of collection.

SUMMARY

1. Under the Medi-Cal regulations, the State can make a claim on a Medi-Cal recipient's estate in order to recover the cost of the Medi-Cal benefits provided. The rule is that the State can collect the lesser of the following:

   A) the cost of the Medi-Cal benefits provided, or

   B) the value of the ill spouse's estate at the time of death. In either case, the State cannot make a claim on the estate until the surviving spouse has died.

2. The method for calculating the amount of the estate claim is as follows:

   Step One: Determine the cost to the State of the Medi-Cal benefits provided.

   Step Two: Determine the value of the Medi-Cal recipient's estate at the time of death.

   Step Three: Compare the two amounts. The lesser number is the amount of the estate claim.

3. Under current practice, Medi-Cal will not make an estate claim on the proceeds of life insurance or annuities.

There are strategies that will enable the ill person to avoid, or at least minimize the effect of, a Medi-Cal estate claim. These are the following strategies:

STRATEGY A: TRANSFER THE ILL SPOUSE'S INTEREST IN THE HOME TO THE WELL SPOUSE.

Transferring the ill spouse's name from the home, prior to the ill spouse's death will protect the home from a Medi-Cal estate claim. Such a transfer will not cause a period of ineligibility for Medi-Cal since Medi-Cal does not penalize gifts of assets between spouses.

STRATEGY B: THE COUPLE TRANSFERS THEIR INTEREST IN THE HOME AND RETAINS A LIFE ESTATE.

Transferring the home and retaining a life estate will at least partially protect the value of the home from the estate claim.

STRATEGY C: DO NOTHING AND APPLY FOR A HARDSHIP WAIVER UPON THE DEATH OF THE SURVIVING SPOUSE.

If an estate claim is made, the recipient of home can apply to the State for a "hardship waiver". The State would then have the option of waiving its right of collection if making a claim would result in financial hardship to the heirs.

SECTION II

PROTECTING THE HOME FROM MEDI-CAL ESTATE CLAIMS
For Single Persons

IF MY LOVED ONE RECEIVES MEDI-CAL BENEFITS AND LATER DIES, CAN THE STATE TAKE THE HOME?

Under the Medi-Cal regulations, the State can make a claim for reimbursement upon the death of the Medi-Cal recipient in order to recover the cost of the Medi-Cal benefits provided. The rule is that the State can collect the lesser of the following:

1) the cost of the Medi-Cal benefits provided, or

2) the value of the ill person's estate at the time of death.

Although the home is an "exempt" asset for the purposes of Medi-Cal eligibility, the home must usually be sold upon the death of the Medi-Cal recipient so that the estate will have enough money to pay the Medi-Cal estate claim. The State, however, will not demand the home itself.

EXAMPLE

Jane, a widow, was in a nursing home and receiving Medi-Cal benefits when she died. She had been receiving Medi-Cal benefits for five years before her death, with a total cost of $100,000 to the State. At the time of death, her only asset was the home worth $85,000. **The amount of the Medi-Cal estate claim?**

The amount of the estate claim is derived as follows:

Step One: Determine the cost to the State of the Medi-Cal benefits provided.

In this example, the cost to the State for Jane's care was $100,000.

Step Two: Determine the value of the Medi-Cal Recipient's Estate at the time of death.

In this example, Jane's home was worth $85,000 at the time of her death.

Step Three: Compare the two amounts. The lesser number is the amount of the estate claim.

In the example, the cost of the Medi-Cal benefits was $100,000. The value of John's estate was $85,000.

Therefore, the amount of the estate claim is **$85,000.**

CAN MEDI-CAL MAKE AN ESTATE CLAIM WHEN MY LOVED ONE HAS A LIVING TRUST WITH NAMED BENEFICIARIES OF THE TRUST PROPERTY?

Yes. Upon the death of the Medi-Cal recipient, the State will make a claim upon the estate. The fact that there is a living trust with named beneficiaries of the trust property is irrelevant to the State. Creditors of the deceased person are entitled to collect against the property in the deceased trust. Therefore, if there is property in the trust at the time of the Medi-Cal recipient's death, the property must be used to satisfy the estate claim. After the estate claim is paid, then any remaining property can be distributed to the named beneficiaries in accordance with the terms written in the trust.

EXAMPLE

Joe Smith, 87, was in a nursing home and received Medi-Cal benefits. He had a living trust which named his two adult children, Joseph Jr. and Samantha, as beneficiaries of the trust property. The only property in the trust was his home, valued at $100,000. Upon Joe's death, the State imposed a $50,000 Medi-Cal estate claim.

The State is entitled to collect $50,000 from the living trust. The fact that Joe's children are the sole beneficiaries to the living trust is irrelevant. Since the State is a creditor, it is entitled to collect the amount owned from the living trust. Since the only property in the living trust was Joe's home, it would be sold, and the estate claim would be satisfied with $50,000 from the proceeds of the sale. The remaining $50,000 would be distributed to Joe's children as the beneficiaries of his trust.

WHAT IF THE TRUST PROPERTY WAS DISTRIBUTED TO THE BENEFICIARIES BEFORE THE STATE COULD COLLECT THE ESTATE CLAIM? CAN THE STATE COLLECT AGAINST THE BENEFICIARIES?

Yes. If the property in the trust is distributed to the beneficiaries prior to satisfying the estate claim, the beneficiaries will be responsible for paying the estate claim, up to the amount of the value of the property that they received from the trust.

EXAMPLE

Joseph Smith, 87, was in a nursing home and received Medi-Cal benefits. He had a living trust which named his two adult children, Joseph Jr. and Samantha, as beneficiaries of the trust property. The only property in the trust was his home, valued at $100,000. Upon Joe's death, the trust distributed the home to Joe's beneficiaries: Joseph Jr. and Samantha. The next month, the State imposed a $50,000 Medi-Cal estate claim on Joseph's estate.

The State is entitled to collect $50,000 from Joseph Jr. and Samantha. It is up to Joseph Jr. and Samantha as to how they will pay the estate claim. They could sell or borrow on the home the inherited, or they could pay the estate claim out of their own personal funds. The point is that since Joseph's children received the property before the estate claim was paid, the State will hold them responsible for paying the estate claim, up to the value of the property they received.

CAN THE STATE MAKE AN ESTATE CLAIM ON THE VALUE OF THE HOME, IF THE HOME IS OWNED IN "JOINT TENANCY" WITH SOMEONE ELSE?

Yes. However, the amount of the claim cannot exceed the value of the Medi-Cal recipient's interest in the home at the time of death. If a Medi-Cal recipient owns his or her home in "joint tenancy", the State will consider the Medi-Cal recipient as only a partial owner of the home. For example, if a Medi-Cal recipient owns a home in joint tenancy with one other person, Medi-Cal will consider the Medi-Cal recipient as a one-half owner of the home. If the Medi-Cal recipient owns a home in joint tenancy with two other persons, the Medi-Cal recipient will be considered to be a one-third owner in the home. Therefore, upon the death of a Medi-Cal recipient, the State can only make a claim on the value of the Medi-Cal recipient's partial interest in the home.

EXAMPLE

George Johnson, was a Medi-Cal recipient. His only asset was his home, which he owned "in joint tenancy" with his daughter, Caroline. When George died, the home was valued at $100,000.

Upon George's death, Medi-Cal can make an estate claim up to the value of George's one-half ownership interest in the home. In this example, George owns his home in joint tenancy with his daughter; therefore, Medi-Cal will consider George to be a one-half owner of the home. Since the estate claim cannot exceed the value of George's ownership interest in the home, the estate claim cannot exceed $50,000 which represents the value of his one-half ownership interest in the home.

IF A PERSON OWNS A HOME "IN JOINT TENANCY", DOESN'T THE DECEASED OWNER'S INTEREST IN THE PROPERTY AUTOMATICALLY PASS TO THE SURVIVING OWNER?

Yes. However, the surviving owner will be responsible for paying the Medi-Cal estate claim up to the value of the ownership interest he or she received. If a Medi-Cal recipient owns a home as a joint tenant with another person, the Medi-Cal recipient is considered to be a one-half owner of the home. Upon the Medi-Cal recipient's death, his or her one-half interest in the home will automatically pass to the surviving owner. When Medi-Cal imposes an estate claim, the surviving owner will then be responsible for satisfying the amount of the estate claim, up to the value of the ownership interest that he or she received.

EXAMPLE

George Johnson, was a Medi-Cal recipient. His only asset was his home which he owned "in joint tenancy" with his daughter, Caroline. When George died, the home was valued at $100,000. His one-half ownership interest in the home automatically passed to his daughter, the surviving joint owner.

Since Caroline received George's ownership interest upon his death, she is responsible for paying the amount of any Medi-Cal estate claim, up to the value of the $50,000 ownership interest she received.

CAN THE STATE PLACE A LIEN ON THE HOME?

If the Medi-Cal recipient intends to return to the home, the State cannot place a lien on the home. Upon the death of the Medi-Cal recipient, the State may place a lien on the home for the amount of the estate claim.

ARE LIFE INSURANCE AND ANNUITIES PROTECTED FROM MEDI-CAL ESTATE CLAIMS?

Yes. Under current practice, Medi-Cal will not make an estate claim on the proceeds of life insurance or annuities, although it has a legal right to do so.

ARE THERE ANY CIRCUMSTANCES IN WHICH THE STATE CANNOT MAKE AN ESTATE CLAIM?

Yes. There are two circumstances in which the State cannot make an estate claim. The first is when the heir or beneficiary of the estate is a minor child of the deceased Medi-Cal recipient. A minor is considered a person under the age of twenty-one. The other circumstance is when the heir or beneficiary is an adult child of the deceased Medi-Cal recipient who is both permanently and totally disabled.

WHEN IS A PERSON PERMANENTLY AND TOTALLY DISABLED FOR THE PURPOSE OF BEING EXEMPTED FROM AN ESTATE CLAIM?

The Medi-Cal regulations do not specifically define "permanently and totally disabled." However, if the adult child whose sole source of income is either SSI (Supplemental Security Income) or Social Security Disability, he or she is likely to qualify for the estate claim exemption.

IS THERE ANY WAY I CAN PROTECT THE VALUE OF MY LOVED ONE'S HOME FROM A MEDI-CAL ESTATE CLAIM?

Yes. There are strategies that will enable the ill person to avoid, or at least minimize the effect of, a Medi-Cal estate claim. These are the following strategies.

STRATEGY A

TRANSFER THE ILL PERSON'S INTEREST IN THE HOME

As previously stated, under the Medi-Cal regulations, the amount of the estate claim will be the lesser of the following:

1) the cost of the Medi-Cal benefits provided, or

2) the value of the Medi-Cal recipient's estate at the time of death.

Therefore, the ill person can transfer his or her home so that the value of the estate will be minimal at the time of death. This value will be the maximum amount that the State can collect from the Medi-Cal recipient's estate. Thus, transferring the home **prior to death** will protect the home from a Medi-Cal estate claim.

BUT IF MY LOVED ONE TRANSFERS THE HOME, DOESN'T THIS TRANSFER CAUSE A PERIOD OF INELIGIBILITY?

Under the Medi-Cal regulations, transfers of "exempt" assets do not result in a period of ineligibility. Since the home is an exempt asset (because your loved one stated on the Medi-Cal application that he or she intends to return home), transferring the home will not adversely affect the ill person's Medi-Cal eligibility. Therefore, Medi-Cal will not impose a period of ineligibility upon the transfer of the home. However, **Medi-Cal will require the recipients of the home to sign an affidavit saying that the Medi-Cal recipient can return to the home whenever he or she wishes and it is medically feasible for him or her to do so** (See the end of Chapter 4 for an example of an Affidavit and Appendix IV for an Affidavit form you can use).

WHAT CAN I DO IF MY LOVED ONE LACKS CAPACITY TO TRANSFER THE HOME?

An ill person cannot legally transfer the home if he or she lacks sufficient mental capacity to sign a deed. If the ill person lacks sufficient capacity to sign a deed, there are several possible alternatives:

1) **The Living Trust**
   If your loved one has a living trust, the trust may give the trustee the necessary legal authority to transfer the home. The attorney who drafted the trust should be consulted.

2) **Durable Power of Attorney for Financial Management**
   If your loved one has signed a Durable Power of Attorney for Financial Management, this document may provide the agent with the necessary legal authority to transfer the home. The attorney who drafted the Durable Power of Attorney for Financial Management should be consulted. (See Forms in Appendix IV)

3) Conservatorship

If your loved one is under a conservatorship, the appointed conservator may have the legal authority to transfer the ill person's interest in the home. However, such transfers usually require the conservator to obtain special permission from the Court having jurisdiction over the conservatorship. The attorney representing either the conservator or the conservatee should be consulted.

STRATEGY B

TRANSFER THE HOME AND RETAIN A LIFE ESTATE

†Note: As in the previous strategy, your loved one will need to have sufficient mental capacity to transfer their interest in their home, even if he or she is retaining a life estate. Also, if this strategy is used, it is suggested that the recipients of the home sign an affidavit stating that the ill person can return home whenever he or she wishes and it is medically feasible to do so. (See Affidavit in the Appendix).

Transferring the home and retaining a life estate will at least partially protect the value of the home from the estate claim. A life estate is an interest in real estate that allows the holder of the life estate, known a the life tenant, the right to occupy the property for the remainder of his or her life. Upon the death of the life tenant, the life estate is terminated and the actual owner of the property then receives the right to occupy the property.

Transferring the home and retaining a life estate will at least partially protect the value of the home from the estate claim because only the actual value of the life estate is subject to the estate claim. Moreover, the State is unlikely to enforce an estate against the value of a life estate because of the difficulty in placing an actual value on a life estate.

Nevertheless, the State retains a right to collect against the Medi-Cal recipient's share in the life estate, for this reason, this strategy does not fully protect the value of the home as effectively as a complete transfer of the home.†

STRATEGY C

DO NOTHING AND APPLY FOR A HARDSHIP WAIVER UPON DEATH OF THE MEDI-CAL RECIPIENT

If the Medi-Cal recipient owned the home at the time of death, the value of his or her share in the property would be subject to an estate claim to reimburse the cost of the Medi-Cal benefits provided.

However, the recipient of the home can apply to Medi-Cal for a "hardship waiver". This waiver asks the State of California to waive its right to make an estate claim because it would result in significant financial hardship to the heirs. The State will also consider other factors in deciding whether to waive the estate claim such as the delayed institutionalization of the ill person because of care provided by the heirs. The State would then have the option of collecting against the estate or waiving its right of collection.

SUMMARY

1. Under the Medi-Cal regulations, the State can make a claim for reimbursement upon the death of the Medi-Cal recipient. The rule is that the State can collect the lesser of the following:

    A) the cost of the Medi-Cal benefits provided, or

    B) the value of the ill person's estate at the time of death.

2. The method of determining the amount of the estate claim is as follows:

    Step One: Determine the cost to the State of the Medi-Cal benefits provided.

    Step Two: Determine the value of the Medi-Cal recipient's estate at the time of death.

    Step Three: Compare the two amounts. The lesser number is the amount of the estate claim.

3. Under current practice, Medi-Cal will not make an estate claim on the proceeds of life insurance or annuities.

There are strategies that will enable the ill person to avoid, or at least minimize the effect of, a Medi-Cal estate claim. These are the following strategies.

STRATEGY A: TRANSFER THE HOME OUT OF THE MEDI-CAL RECIPIENT'S ESTATE.

1. Transferring the home out of the Medi-Cal recipients estate prior to death will protect the home from a Medi-Cal estate claim. In addition, transferring the home will not cause a period of ineligibility as long as the recipients of the home sign an affidavit saying that the Medi-Cal recipient can return to the home whenever he or she wishes and it is medically feasible for him or her to do so. (See **Appendix IV for a sample Affidavit form**).

2. If the ill person lacks sufficient capacity to sign a deed, a caregiver could have the legal authority to sign a deed on behalf of their loved one. This legal authority could exist if there is a Living Trust, a Durable Power of Attorney for Financial Management, or a Conservatorship.

STRATEGY B: TRANSFER THE HOME AND RETAIN A LIFE ESTATE.

Transferring the home and retaining a life estate will at least partially protect the value of the home from the estate claim.

STRATEGY C: DO NOTHING AND APPLY FOR A HARDSHIP WAIVER UPON THE DEATH OF THE MEDI-CAL RECIPIENT.

If an estate claim is made, the recipient of the home can apply to the State for a "hardship waiver". The State would then have the option of waiving its right of collection if making a claim would result in financial hardship to the heirs.

Sample Affidavit Below is a sample affidavit the recipient of the home would complete, notarize and turn into the Medi-Cal Eligibility Worker upon the transfer of the home. An Affidavit form for your use is located in Appendix IV.

1. **COUNTY WHERE AFFIDAVIT IS TO BE FILED**
2. **NAME OF RECIPIENT OF PROPERTY**
3. **NAME OF MEDI-CAL RECIPIENT**
4. **ADDRESS/CITY OF PRINCIPAL RESIDENCE**
5. **NAME OF MEDI-CAL RECIPIENT**
6. **DAY/MONTH/YEAR OF LEAVING HOME**
7. **NAME OF CARE FACILITY**
8. **ADDRESS/CITY OF CARE FACILITY**
9. **HIS/HER/NAME OF MEDI-CAL RECIPIENT**

10. **HE/SHE/NAME OF MEDI-CAL RECIPIENT**
11. **DAY/MONTH/YEAR OF SIGNING**
12. **SIGNATURE OF RECIPIENT OF THE PROPERTY**
13. **COUNTY OF NOTARY PUBLIC**
14. **DAY/MONTH/YEAR OF NOTARY**
15. **NAME OF NOTARY PUBLIC**
16. **NAME OF RECIPIENT APPEARING BEFORE NOTARY**
17. **NOTARY SIGNATURE**
18. **NOTARY SEAL**

AFFIDAVIT

STATE OF CALIFORNIA)
COUNTY OF _____ -1- ___)

I, _____ -2- _____, declare that:

1. I have personal knowledge of the facts herein contained and if called as a witness to testify to such facts, I can competently do so.

2. _____ -3- _____ owned his home and principal residence. This principal residence is located _____ -4- _____, _____ -4- _____, California. _____ -5- _____ lived in that home until _____, -6-, _____.

3. _____ -5- _____ is currently residing at _____ -7- _____ located at _____ -8- _____, _____ -8- _____, California. However, _____ -5- _____ intends to return home based on my personal knowledge of ___ -9- ___ desire to return home if and when _____ -10- _____ is medically able to return home.

4. Consequently, the principle residence, located at _____ -4- _____, _____ -4- _____, California is, and continues to be an exempt asset. I now have an ownership interest in the residence, and I will maintain the home for _____ -5- _____. _____ -5- _____ will be permitted to return to live at the home whenever _____ -10- _____ wishes and it is medically feasible to do so.

I declare under the penalty of perjury under the laws of the State of California that the foregoing is true and correct and that this Affidavit was executed on the ___ -11- ___ day of _____ -11- , -11- .

_____ -2- _____
RECIPIENT OF THE PROPERTY

ACKNOWLEDGEMENT

STATE OF CALIFORNIA)
COUNTY OF _____ -13- ___)

On _____ -14-, _____, before me, _____ -15- _____, Notary Public, personally appeared _____ -16- _____, personally known to me-or-proved to me on the basis of satisfactory evidence to be the person(s) whose name(s) is/are subscribed to the within instrument and acknowledged to me that he/she/they executed the same in his/her/their authorized capacity(ies), and that by his/her/their signature(s) on the instrument the person(s), or the entity upon behalf of which the person(s) acted, executed the instrument.

WITNESS my hand and official seal.

_____ -17- _____   -18-

CHAPTER 5

THE MEDI-CAL INCOME RULES

This Chapter covers the following topics:

Income Limits for the Medi-Cal recipient

Income Limits for the Well Spouse

Share of Cost

The "Name on the Instrument" Rule

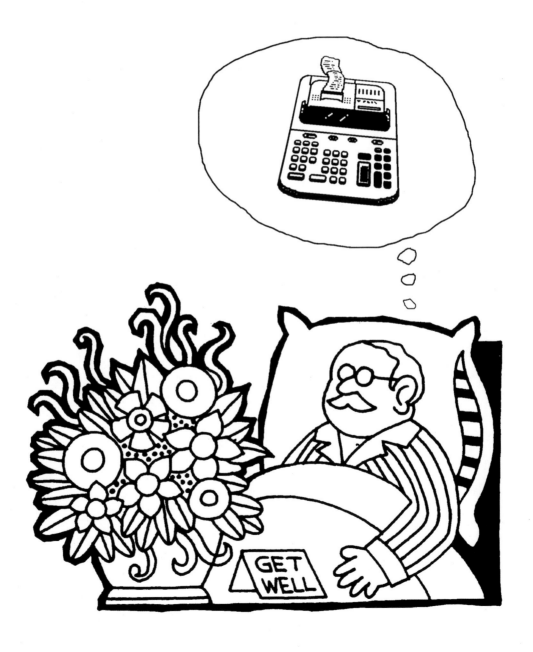

SECTION I

THE MEDI-CAL INCOME RULES For Married Persons

WHAT DOES MEDI-CAL CONSIDER AS "INCOME?"

For Medi-Cal purposes, "income" is money received on a regular basis that has not been in the possession of the Medi-Cal recipient for more than thirty days. Examples of income include Social Security payments, pension payments, IRA distributions, stock dividends, and rent. To be characterized as income, the money must be distributed to either the couple or one of the spouses. For example, interest earned on a Certificate of Deposit would **not** be characterized as income if it merely accumulated in the CD. For the interest to be characterized as "income," the interest payment must be sent to either the couple or one of the spouses.

HOW MUCH OF THE HOUSEHOLD INCOME CAN THE WELL SPOUSE KEEP ONCE THE ILL SPOUSE BEGINS RECEIVING MEDI-CAL BENEFITS?

The current Medi-Cal rules are designed to provide the well spouse with sufficient income (and assets) to have a comfortable standard of living—thus avoiding impoverishment. The monthly amount of income that the well spouse is allowed to keep is known as the "Monthly Minimum Maintenance Needs Allowance" (MMMNA). In 1999, the MMMNA for the well spouse is $2,049 of the household income. As a Medi-Cal recipient, the ill spouse will be allowed to keep only $35.00 per month of his or her income.

WHAT ARE THE CONSEQUENCES IF THE COUPLE HAS EXCESS INCOME? WOULD THE EXCESS INCOME DISQUALIFY THE ILL SPOUSE FROM RECEIVING MEDI-CAL BENEFITS?

How much income the couple receives does not affect or determine the ill spouse's Medi-Cal eligibility. **Any excess income that the couple receives will constitute the ill spouse's monthly "share of cost". This is the amount that the couple will pay directly to the nursing home.** Each month, the well spouse will receive a notice from Medi-Cal which states the amount of the share of cost for the ill spouse. The share of cost is paid directly to the nursing home. Medi-Cal will cover the remaining cost of care.

EXAMPLE

John and Mary are married. John is in a nursing home. He has been determined eligible to receive Medi-Cal benefits. He receives a pension and social security payments which collectively amount to $2,000 per month. Mary receives $500 per month in Social Security. Their combined household income is $2,500 per month.

As the ill spouse, John will be allowed to keep only $35.00 per month of his income. In addition, Medi-Cal will allow Mary (the well spouse) to keep enough of John's income to bring her up to the $2,049 per month level (which is her MMMNA for 1999).

The remaining $446 per month of the household income will constitute John's "share of cost." Mary will pay $446 directly to the nursing home each month for John's nursing home care. Medi-Cal will pay the remaining cost.

IS THERE ANY WAY TO REDUCE THE SHARE OF COST?

The share of cost can be reduced by the amount of any medical insurance premiums and unpaid medical bills incurred by the ill spouse. This rule allows persons receiving Medi-Cal benefits to pay their health insurance premiums and outstanding medical bills without simultaneously having to pay for their nursing home care.

EXAMPLE

John and Mary are a married couple. John is a nursing home patient and receives Medi-Cal benefits. His share of cost is $1,000 per month. However, before John's entry into the nursing home, he incurred a medical bill of $12,000, which he has not yet paid. If John or Mary notifies Medi-Cal of this $12,000 unpaid medical bill, Medi-Cal will suspend John's obligation to pay his share of cost for twelve months. The purpose of the twelve-suspension is to allow the couple to use the $1,000 per month share of cost to pay the unpaid medical bills.

WHAT IS THE "NAME ON THE INSTRUMENT" RULE?

The "name on the instrument" rule allows the well spouse to keep all the income he or she receives in his or her name only. Under this rule, there is no limit to the amount of monthly income that the well spouse can keep, if the check is in the well spouse's name only. Consequently, this rule makes it possible for the well spouse to retain an income level that even exceeds the MMMNA of $2,049.

EXAMPLE

David and Jane are married. David receives $3,000 per month in pension and social security payments. Jane receives $500 per month. Jane is in a nursing home and receives Medi-Cal benefits.

Under the "Name On The Instrument Rule," Medi-Cal will allow David (the well spouse) to keep all of the income he receives in his name only—even if it exceeds the MMMNA of $2,049 per month.

Thus, he will be allowed to keep all $3,000 of his income. Jane will be allowed to keep $35.00 per month of income in her name. The additional $465 per month she receives is her share of cost, which will be paid directly to the nursing home.

SUMMARY

1   For Medi-Cal purposes, "income" is money received on a regular basis that has not been in the possession of the Medi-Cal recipient for more than thirty days. Examples of income include Social Security payments, pension payments, IRA distributions, stock dividends, and rent.

2   The monthly amount of income that the well spouse is allowed to keep is known as the "Monthly Minimum Maintenance Needs Allowance" (MMMNA). In 1999, the MMMNA for the well spouse is $2,049 of the household income. As a Medi-Cal recipient, the ill spouse will be allowed to keep only $35.00 per month of his or her income.

3   The level of income that the couple receives does not affect or determine the ill spouse's Medi-Cal eligibility. Any excess income that the couple receives above their MMMNA (Monthly Minimum Maintenance Needs Allowance) will constitute the ill spouse's monthly "share of cost". This is the amount that the couple will pay directly to the nursing home.

4   The share of cost can be reduced by the amount of any unpaid medical bills incurred by the ill spouse. This rule allows persons receiving Medi-Cal benefits to pay their outstanding medical bills without simultaneously having to pay for their nursing home care.

5   The "Name On The Instrument Rule" rule allows the well spouse to keep all the income he or she receives in his or her name only. Under this rule, there is no limit to the amount of monthly income that the well spouse can keep as long as the income received is only in the name of the well spouse.

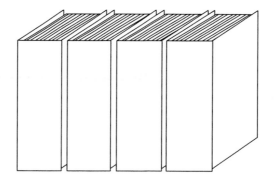

SECTION II

THE MEDI-CAL INCOME RULES FOR SINGLE PERSONS

WHAT DOES MEDI-CAL CONSIDER AS "INCOME"?

Income is money received on a regular basis that has not been in the possession of the Medi-Cal applicant for more than thirty days. Examples of "income" include Social Security payments, pensions, IRA distributions, stock and mutual fund dividends, and rent received. To be characterized as income, the money must actually be distributed to your loved one. For example, interest earned on a Certificate of Deposit would not be characterized as income if it merely accumulated in the CD. For the interest payment to be characterized as "income," it must be sent to your loved one.

DOES THE LEVEL OF INCOME MY LOVED ONE RECEIVES AFFECT HIS MEDI-CAL ELIGIBILITY?

No. The level of income your loved one receives does not affect or determine his or her Medi-Cal eligibility. Once your loved one is receiving Medi-Cal, he will be allowed him to keep only $35.00 per month of his income. However, the excess income he receives will not make him ineligible for Medi-Cal. Any excess monthly income received by the ill person will have to be used to pay for the cost of his nursing home care. This excess income will constitute the Medi-Cal recipient's monthly "share of cost". The ill person will receive a monthly notice from Medi-Cal that will state the amount of the share of cost. Once the share of cost is paid, Medi-Cal will cover the remaining cost of care.

EXAMPLE

John is in a nursing home and receives Medi-Cal benefits. He receives a pension and social security payments of $1,500 per month. Medi-Cal will allow John to keep only $35.00 per month of his income. The $1,465 per month of excess income received by John constitutes his share of cost. Medi-Cal will pay the remaining cost of John's care.

IS THERE ANY WAY TO REDUCE THE SHARE OF COST?

The share of cost will be reduced by any health insurance premiums and any unpaid medical bills incurred by your loved one. This rule allows persons receiving Medi-Cal benefits to pay their health insurance premiums and outstanding medical bills without simultaneously having to pay for their nursing home care.

EXAMPLE

John is in a nursing home. He receives Medi-Cal benefits and his share of cost is $1,000 per month. However, before John entering a nursing home, he had incurred $3,000 in medical bills, which had not been paid. If John notifies Medi-Cal of the $3,000 unpaid medical bill, Medi-Cal will suspend John's obligation to pay the share of cost for three months. This allows John to divert the $1,000 per month share of cost to pay the unpaid balance for his home care.

IN ADDITION TO THE $35.00 ALLOWANCE, DOES MEDI-CAL ALLOW THE ILL PERSON TO RETAIN ENOUGH INCOME TO PAY THEIR PROPERTY TAXES AND GENERAL EXPENSES FOR THE UPKEEP OF THE HOME?

As previously stated, Medi-Cal allows the ill person to retain their home indefinitely as long as he or she intends return home. However, Medi-Cal will only allow the ill person an allowance for property taxes and other home-related expenses if a doctor states that he or she will return home within six months of applying for Medi-Cal. If this doctor's statement is obtained, then Medi-Cal will grant a six month one- time only upkeep allowance for maintaining the home.

Therefore, if the ill person does not return home within six months, he or she will forever lose the upkeep allowance, even if the doctor signs another statement that the ill person will return home within six months.

SUMMARY

1. Income is money received on a regular basis that has not been in the possession of the Medi-Cal applicant for more than thirty days. Examples of "income" include Social Security payments, pensions, IRA distributions, stock and mutual fund dividends, and rent received.

2. Once your loved one is receiving Medi-Cal benefits, Medi-Cal will allow him to keep only $35.00 per month of his income. Any excess income received by the ill person will have to be used to pay for the cost of his nursing home care. This excess income constitutes the Medi-Cal recipient's "share of cost." The level of income your loved one receives does not determine his or her Medi-Cal eligibility it only determines the extent to which your loved one has a share of cost.

3. The share of cost will be reduced by any unpaid medical bills incurred by your loved one. This rule allows persons receiving Medi-Cal benefits to pay their outstanding medical bills without simultaneously having to pay for their nursing home care.

4. Medi-Cal will allow the ill person a six month, one time only allowance for the upkeep and maintenance of the home, including the payment of property taxes, if a doctor states that the ill person will return home within six months of applying for Medi-Cal.

CHAPTER 6

FREQUENTLY ASKED QUESTIONS

This chapter covers the following topics:

Living Trusts

Cash Transfers

After-acquired Property

Fair Hearings

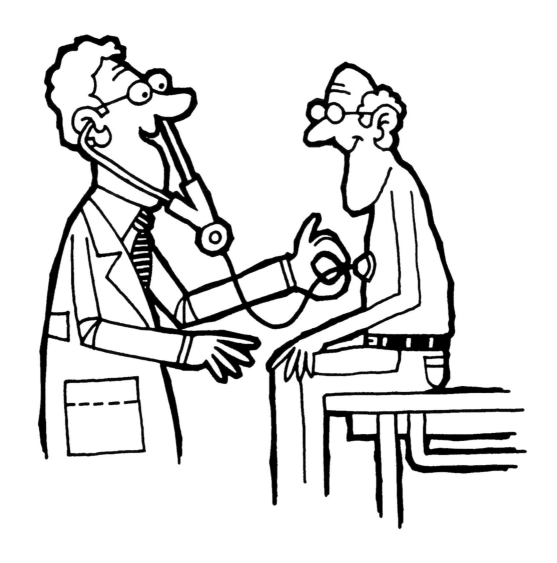

SECTION I

FREQUENTLY ASKED QUESTIONS FOR MARRIED PERSONS

LIVING TRUSTS

DOES TRANSFERRING PROPERTY INTO A LIVING TRUST PROTECT IT FROM BEING COUNTED BY MEDI-CAL?

No. Living trusts are trusts that are created and funded by the couple during their lifetime. The There are two basic types of living trusts: 1) revocable living trusts; and 2) irrevocable living trusts. Transferring the couple's property into their revocable or irrevocable living trust does not make these assets exempt in determining an ill spouse's Medi-Cal eligibility. However, exempt assets placed in a living trust will continue to be exempt from consideration in determining an ill spouse's Medi-Cal eligibility.

CASH TRANSFERS

MY PARENTS TRANSFERRED CASH BEFORE THEY KNEW ABOUT THE MEDI-CAL ELIGIBILITY CONSEQUENCES OF MAKING GIFTS. WHAT CAN BE DONE TO MINIMIZE OR AVOID THESE CONSEQUENCES?

There are several possibilities to avoid or minimize any adverse consequences on Medi-Cal eligibility due to the transfer of cash.

A. RE-ACQUIRE THE CASH

If the couple has transferred cash, but the cash has been returned, Medi-Cal will not impose a period of ineligibility. For example, if a couple transferred $12,000 to their adult child, this transfer would trigger a three-month period of ineligibility. However, Medi-Cal would terminate this period of ineligibility if the person returned the funds. The advantage of this option is that it would eliminate the initial period of ineligibility caused by the gift. However, the disadvantage with this option is that the value of any non-exempt assets returned would be counted in determining the ill spouse's Medi-Cal eligibility.

B. DO NOTHING

The advantage of this option is that transferring the asset(s) effectively reduces the value of the couple's countable assets. The second advantage of the transfer is that it allows the recipient of the asset to retain it for safekeeping. Although the cash transfer results in a period of ineligibility, the transferred funds could be used to pay for the cost of the ill spouse's nursing home care during this period. Any additional cash could continue to be held for "safe keeping" by the recipient of the cash.

AFTER-ACQUIRED PROPERTY

WHAT IF THE WELL SPOUSE ACQUIRES ADDITIONAL PROPERTY AFTER THE ILL SPOUSE IS RECEIVING MEDI-CAL BENEFITS? WILL THIS ADDITIONAL PROPERTY AFFECT THE ILL SPOUSE'S MEDI-CAL ELIGIBILITY?

No, if the ill spouse's name does not appear on the newly acquired property. This is known as the After-Acquired property rule. It essentially states that **after the ill spouse begins receiving Medi-Cal benefits, there is no limit on the value of property the well spouse can later acquire as long as the ill spouse's name is not on the newly-acquired property.**

The Medi-Cal eligibility limit for a married person is $83,960 in 1999. Once the ill spouse is determined eligible for Medi-Cal benefits, the couple will have approximately ninety days to transfer all non-exempt assets (except for $2,000) out of the ill spouse's name, and into the name of the well spouse. This $2,000 amount is called the ill spouse's "property reserve". The $80,760 retained by the well spouse is called the "Community Spouse Resources Allowance (CSRA).

While the spouse is receiving Medi-Cal, he or she cannot have assets which exceed their property reserve. However, assets acquired by the well spouse will not affect the ill spouse's Medi-Cal eligibility **as long as the ill spouse's name is not on the newly-acquired property.** Again, this rule only applies AFTER the ill spouse begins receiving Medi-Cal.

MY WIFE IS IN A NURSING HOME AND RECEIVES MEDI-CAL BENEFITS. IN OUR WILLS, MY WIFE AND I EACH LEAVE EVERYTHING TO THE OTHER. IF I DIE BEFORE SHE DOES, COULD SHE LOSE HER MEDI-CAL ELIGIBILITY AS A RESULT OF PROPERTY SHE WOULD INHERIT FROM ME?

Yes. Any additional non-exempt (countable) assets received by the ill spouse in excess of her $2,000 property reserve will make her ineligible for Medi-Cal benefits. For this reason, the well spouse should consider altering his Will so that the spouse receiving Medi-Cal benefits is disinherited. If the Will disinherits the ill spouse, she would not receive property that could adversely affect her Medi-Cal eligibility.

FAIR HEARINGS

MY HUSBAND'S APPLICATION FOR MEDI-CAL BENEFITS WAS DENIED. CAN WE APPEAL THIS DECISION?

Yes. If an ill spouse's Medi-Cal application is denied, the couple can appeal the denial by requesting a fair hearing. The couple's right to a fair hearing is guaranteed by the due process clause of the federal and state constitutions. If the couples receive an unfavorable decision, the welfare department will send a "Notice of Action". This notice informs the denied applicant of the right to a fair hearing, and states the procedure for requesting a hearing.

WHAT IS THE DEADLINE FOR APPEALING A DENIAL OF MEDI-CAL BENEFITS?

The ill spouse's representative, must request a fair hearing within ninety days of receiving the Notice of Action.

WHAT HAPPENS AT A FAIR HEARING?

At the hearing, each side presents evidence to an Administrative Law Judge. The couple can represent themselves, or they can be represented by an attorney, paralegal, or even a friend. The county's welfare department, which administers the Medi-Cal program, will not be represented by an attorney.

A hearing is much less formal than an actual trial. The hearing is held in a small room at the welfare department, and both sides usually sit at the same table. The ill spouse's representative will first present the Medi-Cal applicant's side of the case to the judge, followed by the county's representative. The representatives on both sides can submit a written argument to the judge, present witnesses under oath, and submit any relevant documents such as deeds, passbook accounts, etc. In fact, the county is required to submit a "Position Statement". In addition, the judge will ask questions that he or she think are important to decide.

WHAT IS A "POSITION STATEMENT"

In a fair hearing, the county will submit its "position statement" to the judge. The county's position statement states its version of the facts, its reason for denying the application, and cites the regulations that support its position. The ill spouse's representative has the right to obtain this position paper three days before the hearing. Reviewing the county's position before the hearing could be extremely useful in preparing the case for the ill spouse. The ill spouse's representative can also prepare a position paper to submit to the judge, but this is not required. If the ill spouse's representative does prepare a position statement, he or she does not have to submit it to the county before the hearing. However, at the hearing, the ill spouse's representative should give a copy of the position statement to the county's representative.

UNDER WHAT CIRCUMSTANCES CAN THE ILL SPOUSE REQUEST A FAIR HEARING?

The ill spouse has a right to a fair hearing any time the county's welfare department denies him or her a benefit. For example, the ill spouse can request a fair hearing if his or her application for Medi-Cal benefits is denied. In addition, the ill spouse can request a hearing if the Welfare Department determines that he or she should pay a greater share of cost than they must pay. The ill spouse can even request a fair hearing if the county welfare department takes longer than forty-five days to approve or deny the application for Medi-Cal benefits.

SUMMARY

LIVING TRUSTS

Placing the couple's assets into a living trust owned by the couple does not insulate the value of these assets from being counted in determining Medi-Cal eligibility. Medi-Cal will count the value of any assets in a living trust that is owned by the couple, unless the asset is exempt.

TRANSFERS OF CASH AND/OR SECURITIES

If the couple made a gift of cash and/or securities and but was unaware of the consequences to the ill spouse's Medi-Cal eligibility, the couple can do the following:

A. RE-ACQUIRE THE CASH

If the couple person has transferred cash, but the cash has been returned, Medi-Cal will not impose a period of ineligibility.

B. DO NOTHING

The advantage of this option is that transferring the asset(s) effectively reduces the value of the couple's countable assets. The second advantage of the transfer is that it allows the recipient of the asset to retain it for safekeeping.

JOINT BANK ACCOUNTS

As a practical matter, Medi-Cal does not consider the creation of a joint bank accounts as a transfer of assets causing a period of ineligibility. A period of ineligibility would result if the other joint owner of the account withdrew funds and used it for his or her benefit.

JOINT TENANCY IN REAL ESTATE

Creating a joint tenancy on the couple's home by placing another person's name on the deed to the property could be considered a partial gift of the home. However, under the Medi-Cal regulations, this partial gift of the residence will not result in a period of ineligibility if the home was exempt at the time that the joint tenancy was created.

AFTER-ACQUIRED PROPERTY

The After-Acquired Property rule essentially states that **after the ill spouse begins receiving Medi-Cal benefits, there is no limit on the value of property the well spouse can later acquire as long as the ill spouse's name is not on the newly-acquired property.**

Any additional non-exempt assets received by the ill spouse in excess of her $2,000 property property reserve will make him or her ineligible for Medi-Cal benefits. For this reason, it may be advisable for the well spouse to alter his or her Will that the ill spouse receiving Medi-Cal benefits is disinherited.

FAIR HEARINGS

If the ill spouse's Medi-Cal application is denied, she can appeal the denial by requesting a fair hearing. At the hearing, each side presents evidence to an Administrative Law Judge. The Medi-Cal applicant can represent herself or she can be represented by an attorney, paralegal, or even a friend. The ill spouse (or her representative) must request a fair hearing within ninety days of receiving the Notice of Action. The ill spouse has a right to a fair hearing any time the county's welfare department denies him or her a benefit.

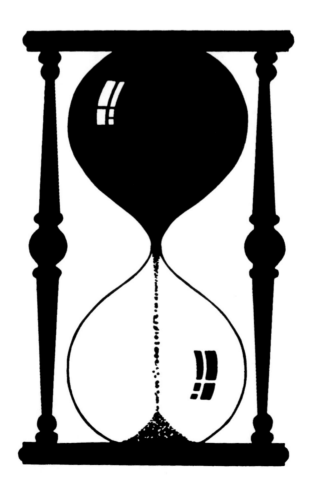

SECTION II

FREQUENTLY ASKED QUESTIONS FOR SINGLE PERSONS

LIVING TRUSTS

DOES TRANSFERRING PROPERTY INTO A REVOCABLE LIVING TRUST PROTECT IT FROM BEING COUNTED BY MEDI-CAL?

No. Living Trusts are trusts that are created and funded by the owner during his or her lifetime. There are two basic types of living trusts: 1) revocable living trusts; and 2) irrevocable living trusts. Placing assets into a revocable or irrevocable living trust does not make these assets exempt. However, exempt assets placed in the living trust will continue to be exempt from consideration in determining Medi-Cal eligibility.

CASH TRANSFERS

MY LOVED ONE TRANSFERRED CASH BEFORE SHE KNEW ABOUT THE MEDI-CAL ELIGIBILITY CONSEQUENCES OF MAKING GIFTS. WHAT CAN BE DONE TO MINIMIZE OR AVOID THESE CONSEQUENCES?

There are several possibilities to avoid or minimize any adverse consequences on Medi-Cal eligibility due to the transfer of cash.

A. RE-ACQUIRE THE CASH

If the ill person has transferred cash, but the cash has been returned, Medi-Cal will not impose a period of ineligibility. For example, if the ill person transferred $12,000 to her adult child, this transfer would trigger a three-month period of ineligibility. However, Medi-Cal would terminate this period of ineligibility if the person returned the funds. The advantage of this option is that it would eliminate the initial period of ineligibility caused by the gift. However, the disadvantage with this option is that the value of any non-exempt assets returned would be counted in determining the ill person's Medi-Cal eligibility.

B. DO NOTHING

The advantage of this option is that transferring the asset(s) effectively reduces the value of the ill person's countable assets. The second advantage of the transfer is that it allows the recipient of the asset to retain it for safekeeping. Although the cash transfer results in a period of ineligibility, the transferred funds could be used to pay for the cost of the ill person's nursing home care during this period. Any additional cash could continue to be held for "safe keeping" by the recipient of the cash.

JOINT ACCOUNTS

DOES THE CREATION OF A JOINT ACCOUNT CAUSE A PERIOD OF INELIGIBILITY?

Elderly persons often create joint tenancy relationships with their family members for two primary purposes: 1) to enable the joint owner to manage the asset in the event he or she becomes ill or incapacitated, and 2) to enable the joint owner to receive full ownership of the asset upon the death of the elderly person, without having to probate the property. The question therefore arises about whether the creation of a joint account would be considered a gift that would cause a period of ineligibility for Medi-Cal benefits.

As a practical matter, Medi-Cal does not consider the creation of a joint account as a transfer of assets causing a period of ineligibility. Medi-Cal is aware that elderly persons often create these accounts for the aforementioned reasons; thus the creation of the joint account, by itself, does not cause a period of ineligibility. However, as a precaution, it is a good idea for the ill person or the other joint account owner to report to Medi-Cal that the funds in the account belong to the ill person applying for Medi-Cal benefits. In fact, Medi-Cal may require the applicant, or applicant's representative sign a statement under penalty of perjury that the funds belong to the ill person.

WHAT ARE THE CONSEQUENCES IF THE OTHER JOINT OWNER ON THE ACCOUNT REMOVES FUNDS FOR HIS OR HER OWN BENEFIT?

A period of ineligibility would result if the other joint owner of the account withdrew funds and used it for his or her benefit. If the funds withdrawn were not used for the benefit of the ill person, Medi-Cal would consider the withdrawal as asset transfer. Such a transfer could result in a period of ineligibility. Consequently, if a person creates a joint account, he or she should keep detailed records of all withdrawals and subsequent expenditures. Such a record would enable Medi-Cal to determine whether such withdrawals were for the ill person's benefit.

DOES THE CREATION OF A JOINT TENANCY ON THE HOME CAUSE A PERIOD OF INELIGIBILITY?

The elderly often create joint tenancy relationships with their family members for two primary purposes: 1) to enable the joint owner to manage the asset in the event they become ill or incapacitated, and 2) to enable the joint owner to receive full ownership of the asset upon the death of the elderly person, without having to probate the home.

Creating a joint tenancy on the ill person's home by placing another person's name on the deed to the property could be considered a gift of one-half the value of the home. However, under the Medi-Cal regulations, this partial gift of the residence will not result in a period of ineligibility if the home was exempt at the time that the joint tenancy was created. As previously stated, gifts of "exempt" assets do not cause a period of ineligibility.

The principal residence was exempt at the time that the joint tenancy was created if: 1) the ill person was living in the home, or 2) the ill person intended to return to the home. If either of these circumstances existed at the time that the joint tenancy was created, Medi-Cal will not impose a period of ineligibility.

As a precaution, the recipient of the joint tenancy interest in the property could sign an affidavit stating that the ill person can return to the home whenever it is medically feasible for him or her to do so. The fact that the ill person is a joint tenant in the home gives him or her the legal right to return to the home. Giving this affidavit to Medi-Cal could avoid unnecessary scrutiny by Medi-Cal with respect to the joint tenancy creation. Such scrutiny could extend the time it takes for Medi-Cal to process the ill person's application.

FAIR HEARINGS

MY MOTHER'S APPLICATION FOR MEDI-CAL BENEFITS WAS DENIED. CAN SHE APPEAL THIS DECISION?
Yes. If the ill person's Medi-Cal application is denied, she can appeal the denial by requesting a fair hearing. The ill person's right to a fair hearing is guaranteed by the due process clause of the federal and state constitutions. If the ill person receives an unfavorable decision on a Medi-Cal application, the county welfare department will send a "Notice of Action". This notice informs the denied applicant of his or her right to a fair hearing, and states the procedure for requesting a hearing.

WHAT IS THE DEADLINE FOR APPEALING A DENIAL OF MEDI-CAL BENEFITS?
The ill person (or her representative) must request a fair hearing within ninety days of receiving the Notice of Action.

WHAT HAPPENS AT A FAIR HEARING?
At the hearing, each side presents evidence to an Administrative Law Judge. The Medi-Cal applicant can represent herself. Alternatively, she can be represented by an attorney, paralegal, or even a friend. The county's welfare department, which administers the Medi-Cal program, will not be represented by an attorney.

A hearing is much less formal than actual trials. The hearing is held in a small room at the welfare department, and both sides usually sit at the same table. The ill person's representative will first present the Medi-Cal applicant's side of the case to the judge, followed by the county's representative. The representatives on both sides can submit a written argument to the judge, present witnesses under oath, and submit any relevant documents such as deeds, passbook accounts, **etc.** In fact, the county is required to submit a "Position Statement". In addition, the judge will ask questions that he or she think are important to reach a decision.

WHAT IS A "POSITION STATEMENT"?

In a fair hearing, the county is required to submit its "position statement" to the judge. The county's position statement states its version of the facts, its reason for denying the application, and cites the regulations that support its position. The ill person's representative has the right to obtain this position statement within three days before the hearing. Reviewing the county's position before the hearing could be extremely useful in preparing the case for the ill person.

The ill person's representative can also prepare a position paper to submit to the judge, but this is not required. If the ill person's representative does prepare a position paper, she does not have to submit it to the county before the hearing. However, at the hearing, the ill person's representative should give a copy of the position paper to the county's representative.

UNDER WHAT CIRCUMSTANCES CAN AN ILL PERSON REQUEST A FAIR HEARING?

The ill person has a right to a fair hearing any time the county's welfare department denies him or her a benefit. For example, the ill person can request a fair hearing if the application for Medi-Cal benefits is denied. In addition, the ill person can request a hearing if the welfare department determines that she should pay a greater share of cost than she expected to pay. The ill person can even request a fair hearing if the county welfare department takes longer than forty-five days to approve or deny the application for Medi-Cal benefits.

SUMMARY

LIVING TRUSTS

Placing the ill person's assets into a revocable or irrevocable living trust owned by the ill person does not insulate the value of these assets from being counted in determining Medi-Cal eligibility. Medi-Cal will count the value of any assets in a revocable living trust that is owned by the ill person, unless the asset is exempt.

TRANSFERS OF CASH AND/OR SECURITIES

If the ill person made a gift of cash and/or securities and but was unaware of the consequences to the ill spouse's Medi-Cal eligibility, he or she can do the following:

A. RE-ACQUIRE THE CASH

If the ill person has transferred cash, but the cash has been returned, Medi-Cal will not impose a period of ineligibility.

B. DO NOTHING

Although the cash transfer would cause a period of ineligibility, the advantage of this option is that transferring the asset(s) effectively reduces the value of the ill person's countable assets. The second advantage of the transfer is that it allows the recipient of the asset to retain it for safekeeping.

JOINT BANK ACCOUNTS

As a practical matter, Medi-Cal does not consider the creation of a joint bank accounts as a transfer of assets causing a period of ineligibility. A period of ineligibility would result if the other joint owner of the account withdrew funds and used it for his or her benefit.

JOINT TENANCY IN REAL ESTATE

Creating a joint tenancy on the ill person's home by placing another person's name on the deed to the property could be considered a partial gift of the home. However, under the Medi-Cal regulations, this partial gift of the residence will not result in a period of ineligibility if the home was exempt at the time that the joint tenancy was created.

FAIR HEARINGS

If the ill person's Medi-Cal application is denied, she can appeal the denial by requesting a fair hearing. At the hearing, each side presents evidence to an Administrative Law Judge. The Medi-Cal applicant can represent herself or she can be represented by an attorney, paralegal, or even a friend. The ill spouse (or her representative) must request a fair hearing within ninety days of receiving the Notice of Action. The ill person has a right to a fair hearing any time the county's welfare department denies him or her a benefit.

APPENDIX

I. A SAMPLE MEDI-CAL PLAN
II. CALCULATING MEDI-CAL ELIGIBILITY
III. ASSET PROTECTION STRATEGIES
IV. LEGAL FORMS

1. Durable Power of Attorney
2. Affidavit
3. Promissory Note

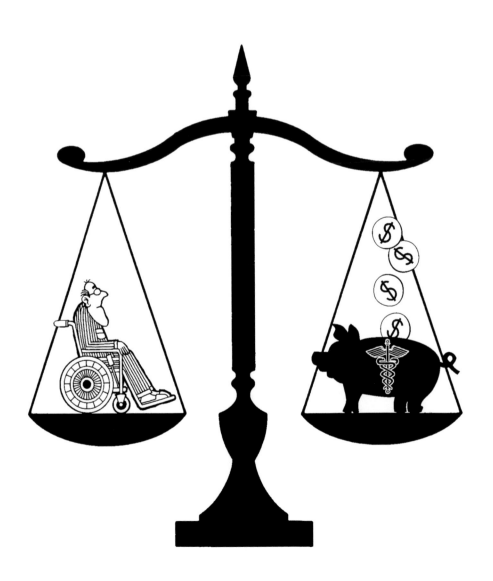

A SAMPLE MEDI-CAL PLAN
FOR MARRIED PERSONS

Bill and Catherine are both 72 years old. They have been married for fifty years. They have one child, Barbara. In their Wills, Bill leaves everything to Catherine, and vice-versa. Both Wills say that if the other spouse dies before the other, then the property is left to their daughter, Barbara.

Last month, Bill has had a stroke and will soon be discharged into a nursing home. The doctor says that Bill may never be able to return home. After learning that Medicare will only pay for a few weeks of Bill's care, Catherine was advised by the social worker at the hospital to apply for Medi-Cal benefits for Bill.

The couple's assets consist of the following:

1.) Their single family home, worth $130,000. Catherine intends to remain in the home but it has a $15,000 mortgage and it needs a new roof that will cost $10,000.

2.) Certificates of deposit worth $150,000;

3.) $20,000 in a savings account.

4.) An 1989 Buick, worth $5,000; and

5.) Bill's $10,000 life insurance policy that has a $5,000 cash surrender value.

STEP #1: DETERMINE IF BILL IS ELIGIBLE FOR MEDI-CAL.

The first step in Bill and Catherine's Medi-Cal Plan involves determining whether Bill is eligible for Medi-Cal. This determination involves a three-step process.

Step 1: List the **types** and **values** of the couple's assets.

Step 2: Categorize the assets as "exempt" or "non-exempt".

Step 3: Add the total value of the non-exempt assets.

TYPE	VALUE	CATEGORY
Family home	$130,000	Exempt
Certificates of deposit	$160,000	Non-exempt
Savings Account	$20,000	Non-exempt
Buick	$5,000	Exempt
Life Insurance	$5,000 cash surrender value	Non-exempt
TOTAL NON-EXEMPT VALUE:	**$185,000**	

Conclusion: Bill is not eligible for Medi-Cal because the couple's assets exceed the $83,960 eligibility limit.

STEP #2: DETERMINE THE AMOUNT OF EXCESS ASSETS

The second step of the Medi-Cal Plan involves determining how much the value of the couple's assets exceeds Medi-Cal limit. The amount of excess assets is determined by taking the amount of the non-exempt (countable assets) and then subtracting the Medi-Cal eligibility limit.

$185,000 (countable assets owned by Bill and Catherine)
– $ 83,960 (Medi-Cal Eligibility limit)
$101,040 in <u>excess cash.</u>

Conclusion: Bill is not eligible for Medi-Cal because the value of the couple's cash assets exceeds the Medi-Cal eligibility limit by $101,040.

STEP #3: USE A COMBINATION OF ASSET PROTECTION STRATEGIES TO PROTECT EXCESS CASH:

The third step in the Medi-Cal Plan is to use a combination of asset protection strategies to protect the excess cash. These are some of the strategies that Bill and Catherine could implement.

PURCHASE EXEMPT ASSETS

Bill and Catherine can use some of the excess cash to purchase exempt assets. In the example, the home exempt because Catherine will continue living in the home. However, the home has a $15,000 mortgage and needs a new roof that will cost $10,000. Consequently, Bill and Catherine could spend $25,000 of the excess cash on the mortgage and home repairs. They could spend additional funds on a burial plots, and revocable and irrevocable burial funds.

PAY OFF DEBTS

Second, Bill and Catherine could pay off outstanding debts such as credit card bills, car loans, or other obligations. Medi-Cal allows either spouse to pay their past and present obligations. There is no penalty for paying the debts of either spouse.

PAY FOR SIX MONTHS OF NURSING HOME CARE

Third, Bill and Catherine could set aside $20,000 to pay privately for Bill's nursing home care. As stated previously, the ability to pay privately for care can significantly increase one's chances of gaining admission into a quality nursing facility. This set aside fund should pay for approximately six months of nursing home care, and Bill and Catherine could use the $20,000 savings account for this specific purpose.

MAKE A $20,000 CASH GIFT TO THEIR DAUGHTER

Fourth, Bill and Catherine can give $20,000 cash gift to Barbara. This gift will reduce their excess cash assets by $20,000. In addition, this gift will allow the Barbara to have this money available to her father in order to pay for items or services that Medi-Cal does not cover. Although this gift will cause a five month period of ineligibility for Bill, according to this Medi-Cal Plan, Catherine will be paying for Bill's care out of their own funds anyway for the next six months. Since the period of ineligibility begins on the date that the gift is made, and since it will only be five months in duration (see Chapter 2 on how to calculate the period of ineligibility). Consequently, the ineligibility period will be over when Bill is ready to convert to Medi-Cal.

PURCHASE AN IRREVOCABLE ANNUITY

Fifth, Bill and Catherine could use the remaining **excess** cash to purchase an irrevocable annuity in Catherine's in name. Monies placed in the irrevocable annuity will not be counted towards Bill's Medi-Cal eligibility as long as it periodically distributes both interest and principal. The annuity would also be exempt if it was purchased in Bill's name. The advantage of purchasing it in Catherine's name is that she will be allowed to keep all distributions from the annuity if the annuity is in her name only (See Chapter 5 discussion on the "name on the instrument rule").

Conclusion: Using the above strategies should make Bill eligible for Medi-Cal benefits, once the $20,000 in private pay set aside funds are exhausted.

STEP #4: TRANSFER BILL'S INTEREST IN THE HOME TO CATHERINE TO PROTECT THE HOME FROM A FUTURE MEDI-CAL ESTATE CLAIM

The fourth step in the Medi-Cal Plan is to transfer Bill's interest in their home to Catherine prior to his death. If the above strategies are implemented, Bill should become eligible for Medi-Cal. However, the State will seek to be repaid for the cost of the Medi-Cal benefits to Bill upon the death of Bill and Catherine. (Medi-Cal does not make an estate claim on the Medi-Cal recipient's death until the death of both spouses). If Bill is in a nursing home for a significant period of time, this estate claim made by Medi-Cal could substantially reduce or even exhaust the entire estate. If there is not sufficient cash in the estate the couple's home will likely be sold and the proceeds used to repay the State for Bill's care. Although, Bill and Catherine intended their only child, Barbara, to inherit the family home, the home may be lost forever as a result of the Medi-Cal estate claim.

In order to protect the value of the home from a Medi-Cal claim, Bill should transfer his interest in the home to Catherine. There is a very practical reason for this strategy. Since the home is valued at $130,000, the value of Bill's _ interest in the home is $65,000. Without the transfer of Bill's _ interest in the home, the $65,000 value of this interest would be subject to the estate claim. However, under the Medi-Cal regulations, the value of Bill's interest in the home will not be subject to a Medi-Cal estate claim **if he does not own the interest at the time of his death.** For this reason, transferring Bill's interest in the home to his wife, Catherine, is an effective strategy for protecting the value of the home from a Medi-Cal estate claim. Finally, the transfer of Bill's interest in the home to Catherine would not cause a period of ineligibility for Bill since transfers between spouses do not create a period of ineligibility.

STEP #5: CHANGE WILL OF WELL SPOUSE TO DISINHERIT SPOUSE RECEIVING MEDI-CAL.

The fifth step in the Medi-Cal Plan involves changing Catherine's Will to disinherit Bill. There is a practical reason for doing this. Under the Medi-Cal regulations, once the ill spouse begins receiving Medi-Cal benefits, he or she will have approximately 90 days to transfer all of the **non-exempt assets**, with the exception of $2,000, out of his or her name and into the name of the well spouse. Thereafter, the ill spouse receiving Medi-Cal cannot have more than $2,000 in their name.

Typically, couples have Wills in which each spouse leaves everything to the surviving spouse. However, if the well spouse dies before the ill spouse receiving Medi-Cal, the ill spouse is likely inherit enough property to cause him or her to exceed their $2,000 Medi-Cal eligibility limit, and therefore lose his or her Medi-Cal benefits.

In order to avoid this situation, Catherine could change her Will so that if she dies before Bill, her daughter would inherit her property. This strategy could avoid a potential loss of Medi-Cal benefits for Bill, while preserving the inheritance for Barbara.

CONCLUSION

If the above strategies are implemented, Bill and Catherine can preserve a substantial portion of their assets, while obtaining Medi-Cal eligibility for Bill. Further, the value of the home will be protected from a Medi-Cal estate claim upon the death of both spouses. Finally, if Catherine should predecease Bill, he will not lose his Medi-Cal eligibility since the change in Catherine's Will leaves everything to Barbara.

The implementation of the above strategies, however, could have tax and estate planning consequences for Bill and Catherine. Consequently, Bill and Catherine should not implement any of these strategies without first consulting a CPA and an attorney knowledgeable in elderlaw and estate planning.

A SAMPLE MEDI-CAL PLAN
FOR A SINGLE PERSON

Sarah is 81 years old. She is a widow who had been married for fifty years before her husband died. She has one child, Carolyn. In her Will, Sarah leaves all of her property to Carolyn. Sarah also has a Durable Power of Attorney for Financial Management and has named Carolyn as the agent to handle her finances.

Sarah is suffering from the latter stages of Alzheimer's disease. Last month the children made the decision, upon the recommendation of Sarah's doctor, to place her in a nursing home. Given the nature of Alzheimer's disease, the doctor says that Sarah is unlikely to ever return home. After learning that Medicare will not pay for her care, Carolyn was advised to apply for Medi-Cal benefits for Sarah.

Sarah's assets consist of the following:

1.) Her single family home, worth 130,000. Sarah intends to return home. It has has a $15,000 mortgage and it needs a new roof that will cost $10,000.

2.) Certificates of deposit worth $100,000;

3.) $20,000 in a checking account,

4.) A 1975 Buick, worth $2,000; and

5.) A $10,000 life insurance policy that has a $5,000 cash surrender value.

STEP #1: DETERMINE IF SARAH IS ELIGIBLE FOR MEDI-CAL.

The first step in Sarah's Medi-Cal Plan involves determining whether she is eligible for Medi-Cal. This determination involves a three-step process.

Step 1: List the **types** and **values** of the person's assets.

Step 2: Categorize the assets as "exempt" or "non-exempt".

Step 3: Add the total value of the non-exempt assets.

TYPE	VALUE	CATEGORY
Home	$130,000	Exempt
Certificates of deposit	$100,000	Non-exempt
Checking Account	$20,000	Non-exempt
Buick	$2,000	Exempt
Life Insurance	$5,000 cash surrender value	Non-exempt
TOTAL NON-EXEMPT VALUE:	**$125,000**	

Conclusion: Sarah is not eligible for Medi-Cal because the value of her non-exempt assets exceed the $2,000 eligibility limit.

STEP #2: DETERMINE THE AMOUNT AND TYPE OF EXCESS ASSETS

The second step of the Medi-Cal Plan involves determining how much the value of Sarah's non-exempt (countable) couple's assets exceeds Medi-Cal limit. The amount of excess assets is determined by taking the amount of the non-exempt (countable assets) and then subtracting the Medi-Cal eligibility limit.

$$\begin{array}{r} \$125,000 \\ -\ \underline{\$\ \ \ 2,000}\ \text{(Medi-Cal Eligibility limit)} \\ \$123,000\ \text{in}\ \underline{\text{excess cash.}} \end{array}$$

Conclusion: Sarah is not eligible for Medi-Cal because the value of her cash assets exceeds the Medi-Cal eligibility limit by $123,000.

STEP #3: USE A COMBINATION OF ASSET PROTECTION STRATEGIES TO PROTECT EXCESS CASH:

The third step in the Medi-Cal Plan is to use a combination of asset protection strategies to protect the excess cash. These are some of the strategies that Carolyn could implement for Sarah:

PURCHASE EXEMPT ASSETS
Carolyn can use some of the excess cash to purchase exempt assets for Sarah. In the example, the home is exempt because Sarah intends to return to the home. However, the home has a $15,000 mortgage and needs a new roof that will cost $10,000. Consequently, Carolyn could spend $25,000 of the excess cash on the mortgage and home repairs. Carolyn could also spend additional funds to purchase a burial plot, and revocable and irrevocable burial funds.

WITHDRAW CASH FROM THE LIFE INSURANCE POLICY AND PAY OFF DEBTS
Second, Carolyn could withdraw cash from the life insurance policy. Sarah has a cash surrender value of $5,000 from the life insurance policy. Since the Medi-Cal eligibility limit is $2,000, it is necessary for Carolyn to withdraw the funds and thus reduce the cash surrender value of the policy if Sarah is to become Medi-Cal eligible.

The funds withdrawn from the policy can be used in a variety of ways. For example, they can be used to pay off Sarah's outstanding debts such as credit card bills, personal loans, or other financial obligations. Medi-Cal allows the ill person to pay their past and present obligations. There is no penalty for paying personal debts. If Sarah had no personal debts, Carolyn can use other strategies mentioned in this plan to use or protect the withdrawn cash.

PAY FOR SIX MONTHS OF NURSING HOME CARE

Third, Carolyn could set aside $20,000 to pay privately for Sarah's nursing home care. As stated previously, the ability to pay privately for care can significantly increase one's chances of gaining admission into a quality nursing facility. This set aside fund should pay for approximately six months of nursing home care and Carolyn and could use the $20,000 in Sarah's checking account for this specific purpose.

MAKE CASH GIFTS TO THE CHILDREN

Fourth, Carolyn can make cash gifts to herself in order to reduce the value of Sarah's excess cash. For example, a gift of $20,000 will reduce Sarah's excess cash by $20,000. In addition, this gift will allow Carolyn to have money available for her mother to pay for items or services that Medi-Cal does not cover.

Although this gift will cause a period of ineligibility for Sarah, according to this Medi-Cal Plan, Sarah will be paying for her care out of their own funds anyway for the next six months. Since the period of ineligibility begins on the date that the gift is made, and since it will only be five months in duration (see Chapter 2 on how to calculate the period of ineligibility), the ineligibility period will be over when Sarah is ready to convert to Medi-Cal.

PURCHASE AN IRREVOCABLE ANNUITY

Fifth, Carolyn could use the remaining **excess** cash to purchase an irrevocable annuity in Sarah's name. Monies placed in the irrevocable annuity will not be counted towards Sarah's Medi-Cal eligibility as long as it periodically distributes both interest and principal.

Conclusion: Using the above strategies should make Sarah eligible for Medi-Cal benefits, once the $20,000 in private pay set aside funds are exhausted.

STEP #4: TRANSFER SARAH'S INTEREST IN THE HOME TO PROTECT THE HOME FROM A FUTURE MEDI-CAL ESTATE CLAIM

The fourth step in the Medi-Cal Plan is to transfer Sarah's interest in the home to Carolyn prior to Sarah's death. If the above strategies are implemented, Sarah should become eligible for Medi-Cal. However, the State will seek to be repaid for the cost of the Medi-Cal benefits to upon her death. If Sarah is in a nursing home for a significant period of time, this estate claim made by Medi-Cal could substantially reduce or even exhaust the entire estate. Since she is only allowed to have two thousand dollars in cash as a Medi-Cal recipient, there will not be sufficient cash in the estate to cover the cost of an estate claim. Consequently, her home will likely be sold and the proceeds used to repay the State for Sarah's care. Although, Sarah intended Carolyn to inherit the family home, the home may be lost forever as a result of the Medi-Cal estate claim.

In order to protect its value from a Medi-Cal estate claim upon her death, Sarah's interest in the home must be transferred out of her name, prior to her death. The value of Sarah's home is $130,000. Under the Medi-Cal regulations, the amount of the estate claim will be the lesser of the following: 1) the cost of the Medi-Cal benefits provided, or 2) the value of the ill person's estate at the time of death. Without the transfer of her interest in the home, the $130,000 value of the home would be subject to the estate claim. However, if Sarah does not own the home at the time of her death, then the value of the home cannot be subject to an estate claim. For this reason, transferring Sarah's interest can be an effective strategy for protecting the value of the home from a Medi-Cal estate claim. Finally, the transfer of Sarah's interest in the home would not cause a period of ineligibility for Sarah as long as the recipient of the home (i.e. Carolyn) signs an affidavit saying that her mother can return to live in the home whenever her return is medically feasible.

CONCLUSION

If the above strategies are implemented, Sarah can preserve a substantial portion of their assets, while obtaining Medi-Cal eligibility. Further, the value of the home will be protected from a Medi-Cal estate claim upon the death of Sarah.

The implementation of the above strategies, however, could have tax and estate planning consequences for Sarah. Consequently, Carolyn should not implement any of these strategies on behalf of Sarah without first consulting a CPA and an attorney knowledgeable in elderlaw and estate planning.

CALCULATING MEDI-CAL ELIGIBILITY
FOR MARRIED PERSONS

Use This Form to Determine Medi-Cal Eligibility For Married Persons.

STEP 1: LIST THE TYPE AND VALUE OF ASSETS OWNED BY EITHER OR BOTH SPOUSES.

STEP 2: CATEGORIZE EACH ASSET AS "EXEMPT OR NON-EXEMPT."

STEP 3: ADD THE TOTAL VALUE OF THE NON-EXEMPT ASSETS.
(The Medi-Cal eligibility limit for Married Persons is $83,960.)

Type	Category	Value
1. Principal Residence	EXEMPT (if spouse lives in the home)	
2. Rental Property	NON-EXEMPT	
3. Savings and Checking Accounts	NON-EXEMPT	
4. Stocks, Bonds, Mutual Funds, Deeds of Trust, Promissory Notes	NON-EXEMPT	
5. Retirement Accounts (IRA's, 401Ks)	EXEMPT (if owned by the at home spouse, or if ill spouse receives a distribution)	
5. Variable Annuities	NON-EXEMPT	
6. Fixed Annuities	EXEMPT (if receiving a distribution)	
7. Whole Life Insurance (cash surrender value)	NON-EXEMPT (if combined face values greater than $1,500)	
8. Personal Jewelry	EXEMPT	
9. Automobile/Household Goods	EXEMPT	
10. Burial Plots, Burial Insurance	EXEMPT	
11. Revocable Burial Fund	EXEMPT (if $1,500 or less)	

Total Value of Non-Exempt Assets:

CALCULATING MEDI-CAL ELIGIBILITY
FOR SINGLE PERSONS

Use This Form to Determine Medi-Cal Eligibility For Single Persons.

STEP 1: LIST THE TYPE AND VALUE OF ASSETS OWNED.

STEP 2: CATEGORIZE EACH ASSET AS "EXEMPT OR NON-EXEMPT."

STEP 3: ADD THE TOTAL VALUE OF THE NON-EXEMPT ASSETS.
(The Medi-Cal eligibility limit for Single Persons is $2,000.)

Type	Category	Value
1. Principal Residence	EXEMPT (if intent to return home)	
2. Rental Property	NON-EXEMPT	
3. Savings and Checking Accounts	NON-EXEMPT	
4. Stocks, Bonds, Mutual Funds, Deeds of Trust, Promissory Notes	NON-EXEMPT	
5. Retirement Accounts (IRA's 401Ks)	EXEMPT (if receiving a distribution)	
6. Variable Annuities	NON-EXEMPT	
7. Fixed Annuities	EXEMPT (if receiving a distribution)	
7. Whole Life Insurance (cash surrender value)	NON-EXEMPT (if combined face values greater than $1,500)	
9. Personal Jewelry (engagement and wedding rings)	EXEMPT	
10. Automobile/Household Goods	EXEMPT	
11. Burial Plots, Burial Insurance	EXEMPT	
12. Revocable Burial Fund	EXEMPT (If $1,500 or less)	

Total Value of Non-Exempt Assets:

ASSET PROTECTION STRATEGIES
FOR MARRIED PERSONS

Check Each Box For Each Strategy Used

STRATEGIES FOR PROTECTING CASH

- ☐ 1. Purchase Exempt Assets (pg. 35)
- ☐ 2. Purchase an Irrevocable Annuity (pg. 36)
- ☐ 3. Transfer Cash and/or Securities (pg. 36)
- ☐ 4. Pay off Debts (Except Medical Bills) (pg. 38)
- ☐ 5. Obtain a Court Order (pg. 39)

STRATEGIES FOR PROTECTING RENTAL PROPERTY

- ☐ 1. Transfer the Rental Property (pg. 40)
- ☐ 2. Borrow on the Rental Property (pg. 42)

STRATEGIES FOR PROTECTING RETIREMENT ACCOUNTS

- ☐ Ill spouse receives periodic distributions from the accounts. (pg. 43)

STRATEGIES FOR PROTECTING CASH VALUE
FROM LIFE INSURANCE

- ☐ Remove the cash from the accounts, and use strategies for protecting cash. (pg. 44)

STRATEGIES FOR PROTECTING THE HOME

- ☐ 1. Transfer home to the well spouse. (pg. 63)
- ☐ 2. Transfer home and retain a life estate. (pg. 65)
- ☐ 3. Do nothing and apply for a hardship waiver upon the death of the surviving spouse. (pg. 65)

ASSET PROTECTION STRATEGIES
FOR SINGLE PERSONS

Check Each Box For Each Strategy Used

STRATEGIES FOR PROTECTING CASH

- ☐ 1. Purchase Exempt Assets (pg. 48)
- ☐ 2. Purchase an Irrevocable Annuity (pg. 49)
- ☐ 3. Transfer Cash and/or Securities (pg. 49)
- ☐ 4. Pay off Debts (Except Medical Bills) (pg. 51)

STRATEGIES FOR PROTECTING RENTAL PROPERTY

- ☐ 1. Transfer the Rental Property (pg. 52)
- ☐ 2. Borrow on the Rental Property (pg. 54)

STRATEGIES FOR PROTECTING RETIREMENT ACCOUNTS

- ☐ Receive periodic distributions from the accounts. (pg. 55)

STRATEGIES FOR PROTECTING CASH VALUE FROM LIFE INSURANCE

- ☐ Remove the cash from the accounts, and use strategies for protecting cash. (pg. 56)

STRATEGIES FOR PROTECTING THE HOME

- ☐ 1. Transfer the ill persons home. (pg. 71)
- ☐ 2. Transfer the ill persons home and the ill person retains a life estate. (pg. 72)
- ☐ 3. Do nothing and apply for a hardship waiver upon the death of the ill person. (pg. 72)

L E G A L   F O R M S   IV

1. Durable Power of Attorney

A Durable Power of Attorney for Financial Management gives caregivers the legal authority to handle financial matters on behalf of their loved one.

2. Affidavit

An Affidavit is a written statement made under penalty of perjury. It has same legal effect as if the person signing the document were testifying in a court of law.

See Chapter 4 Page 74 for Assitance regarding filling out the form

3. Promissory Note

The promissory note should be signed by the person borrowing money as evidence of the legal obligation to repay the money borrowed.

DURABLE POWER OF ATTORNEY

I, _____ ("Principal"), hereby appoint
_____, ("Agent"), as the Principal's true and lawful
attorney-in-fact for the Principal and in the Principal's name, place and stead:

1. To manage, control, lease, sublease, and otherwise act concerning any real property which the Principal may own, collect and receive rents or income therefrom; pay taxes charges, and assessments on the same; repair, maintain, protect, preserve, alter, and improve the same; and do all things necessary or expedient to be done in the Agent's judgment in connection with the property.

2. To manage and control all partnership interests owned by the Principal and to make all decisions the Principal could make as a general partner, limited partner, or both, and to execute all documents required of the Principal as such partner, all to the extent that the Agent's designation for such purposes is allowed by law and is not in contravention of any partnership or other agreement.

3. To purchase, sell, invest, reinvest and generally deal with all stocks, bonds, debentures, warrants, partnership interests, rights, and securities owned by the Principal, including but not limited to any securities described on any exhibit attached to this instrument.

4. To collect and deposit for the benefit of the Principal all debts, interest, dividends or other assets that may be due or belong to the Principal, and to execute and deliver receipts and other discharges therefore; to demand, arbitrate, and pursue litigation on the Principal's behalf concerning all rights and benefits to which the Principal may be entitled; and to compromise, settle, and discharge all such matters as the Agent considers appropriate under the circumstances.

5. To pay any sums of money which may at any time be or become owing from the Principal; to sell, and to adjust and compromise any claims which may be made against the Principal as the Agent considers appropriate under the circumstances.

6. To grant, sell, transfer, disclaim, mortgage, deed in trust, pledge and otherwise deal in all property, real and personal, which the Principal may own, including but not limited to any real property described on any exhibit attached to this instrument including property acquired after execution of this instrument; and to execute any such instruments as the Agent deems proper in conjunction with all matters covered in this paragraph.

7. To prepare and file all income and other federal and state tax returns which the Principal is required to file; to sign the Principal's name; hire preparers and advisors and pay for their services; and to do whatever is necessary to protect the Principal's assets from assessments for income taxes and other taxes for the years 1980 to 2030. The Agent is specifically authorized to receive confidential information; to receive checks in payment of any refund of taxes, penalties, or interest; to execute waivers (including offers of waivers) of restrictions on assessment or collection of tax deficiencies and waivers of notice of disallowance of claims for credit or refund; to execute consents extending the statutory credit or refund; to execute consents extending the statutory period for assessment or collection of taxes; to execute closing agreements under Internal Revenue Code Section 7121, or any successor statute; and to delegate authority or substitute another representative with respect to all above matters.

8. To establish any accounts with any financial institution including but not limited to banks, savings and loans and thrift institutions. The Principal authorizes the Agent to establish any savings, checking and burial accounts or any other accounts the Agent deems necessary with the Principal's assets on such terms as the Agent determines are necessary or proper.

9. To deposit in and draw on any checking, savings, agency, or other accounts which the Principal may have in any banks, savings and loan associations, and any accounts with securities brokers or other commercial institutions, and to establish and terminate all such accounts.

10. To invest and reinvest the Principal's funds in every kind of property, real, personal, or mixed, and every kind of investment, specifically including, but not limited to, corporate obligations of every kind; preferred or common stocks; shares of investment trusts, investment companies, and mutual funds; mortgage participation; that under the circumstances then prevailing (specifically including but not limited to the general economic conditions and the Principal's anticipated needs) persons of skill, prudence, and diligence acting in a similar capacity and familiar with those matters would use in the conduct of an enterprise of a similar character and with similar aims, to attain the Principal's goals; and to consider individual investments as part of an overall plan.

11. To have access to all safe deposit boxes in the Principal's name or to which the Principal is an authorized signatory; to contract with financial institutions for the maintenance and continuation of safe deposit boxes in the Principal's name; to add to and remove the contents of all such safe deposit boxes, and to terminate contracts for all such safe deposit boxes.

12. To bring suit against any bank, savings and loan association, or other person or entity that fails or refuses to honor this power of attorney.

13. To make direct payments to the provider for tuition and medical care for the Principal's issue under Internal Revenue Code Section 2503 (e) or any successor statute, which excludes such payments from gift tax liability.

14. To use any credit cards in the Principal's name to make purchases and to sign charge slips on behalf of the Principal as may be required to use such credit cards; and to close the Principal's charge accounts and terminate the Principal's credit cards under circumstances where the Agent considers such acts to be in the Principal's best interest.

15. To establish any revocable living trusts with the Principal's assets on such terms as the Agent determines are necessary or proper so long as the trust does not materially change the general disposition of the Principal's existing estate plan.

16. To make additions and transfer assets to any existing or future revocable living trusts of which the Principal is the settlor. The Agent is authorized to execute and deliver revocable living trust agreements, to make additions to any existing or future living trusts of which the Principal is the settlor; and to amend or terminate such trusts, so long as such acts do not substantially alter distribution of the Principal's estate during the Principal's lifetime or on the Principal's death, and so long as all such acts do not cause adverse tax consequences for the Principal's estate.

17. Generally to do, execute, and perform any other act, deed, matter, or thing, that in the opinion of the Agent ought to be done, executed, or performed in conjunction with this power of attorney, of every kind and nature, as fully and effectively as the Principal could do if personally present. The enumeration of specific items, acts, rights, or powers in this instrument does not limit or restrict, and is not to be construed or interpreted as limiting or restricting, the general powers granted to the Agent except where powers are expressly restricted.

18. Any third party from whom the Agent may request information, records, or other documents regarding the Principal's personal affairs may release and deliver all such information, records, or documents to the Agent. The Principal hereby waives any privilege that may apply to release of such information, records, or other documents.

19. The Agent's signature under the authority granted in this power of attorney may be accepted by any third party or organization with the same force and effect as if the Principal were personally present and acting on the Principal's own behalf. No person or organization who relies on the Agent's authority under this instrument shall incur any liability to the Principal, the Principal's estate, heirs, successors, or assigns, because of reliance on this instrument.

20. The Principal's estate, heirs, successors, and assigns shall be bound by the Agent's acts under this power of attorney.

21. This power of attorney shall <u>not</u> be affected by the Principal's subsequent disability or incapacity.

22. The Principal hereby ratifies and confirms all that the Agent shall do, or cause to be done, by virtue of this power of attorney.

23. The Principal declares that the Principal understands the importance of this durable power of attorney, recognizes that the Agent is granted broad power to hold, administer and control the Principal's assets. The Principal declares that the Principal understands that when this durable power of Attorney becomes effective, it will continue indefinitely until specifically revoked or terminated by death, even if the Principal later becomes incapacitated.

24. The Agent is authorized to do all things and enter into all transactions necessary to provide for the Principal's personal care, to maintain the Principal's customary standard of living, to provide suitable living quarters for this Principal, and to hire and compensate household, nursing, and other employees as the Agent consider advisable for the Principal's well being. The above shall specifically include but not be limited to the authority to pay the ongoing costs of maintenance of the Principal's present residence, such as interest, taxes, repairs; to procure and pay for clothing, transportation, medicine, medical care, food and other needs; to make arrangements and enter into contracts on behalf of the Principal with hospitals, hospices, nursing homes, convalescent homes, and similar organizations.

25. The Agent is authorized to apply for and make any elections required for payment of governmental, insurance, retirement, or other benefits to which the Principal may be entitled, and to take possession of all such benefits and to distribute such benefits to and for the benefit of the Principal.

26. The Agent is authorized to make gifts on the Principal's behalf to a class composed of the Principal's children, any of their issue, or both to the full extent of the federal annual gift tax exclusion under Internal Revenue Code Section 2503 (b) or any successor statute.

27. The Agent is authorized to engage in any transactions the Agent considers in the Principal's best interest, irrespective of any concurrent interest or benefit to the Agent personally.

28. The Agent is authorized to make photocopies of this instrument and any attached documents as frequently and in such quantity as the Agent deems appropriate. Each photocopy shall have the same force and effect as the original.

30. This power of attorney executed pursuant to the Civil Code of California shall be governed by the laws of the State of California.

31. This power of attorney shall continue after the Principal's incapacity in accordance with its terms.

The Principal hereby guarantees the Agent's signature below.

_____
                          AGENT

If for any reason the Agent is unwilling or unable to continue to serve under this durable power of attorney, _____ shall instead serve as agent. In such case, one of the following documents shall be attached to this durable power of attorney: a resignation or declination to serve signed by the original Agent; a written and signed opinion from a licensed physician that the original Agent is physically or mentally incapable of serving; a certified court order as to the incapacity or inability of the original Agent to serve; or a certified death certificate of the original Agent.

Third parties who deal with the successor Agent shall be entitled to rely on the original power of attorney instrument with any such document attached.

IN WITNESS WHEREOF, the Principal has signed this durable power of attorney on the _____day of _____, _____.

_____
                          PRINCIPAL

ACKNOWLEDGEMENT

STATE OF CALIFORNIA   )
COUNTY OF _____   )

On _____,_____, before me, _____, Notary Public, personally   appeared

_____,
personally known to me-or-proved to me on the basis of satisfactory evidence to be the person(s) whose name(s) is/are subscribed to the within instrument and acknowledged to me that he/she/they executed the same in his/her/their authorized capacity(ies), and that by his/her/their signature(s) on the instrument the person(s), or the entity upon behalf of which the person(s) acted, executed the instrument.

WITNESS my hand and official seal.

_____

AFFIDAVIT

STATE OF CALIFORNIA   )
COUNTY OF _____)

I, _____, declare that:

1. I have personal knowledge of the facts herein contained and if called as a witness to testify to such facts, I can competently do so.

2. _____ owned his home and principal residence. This principal residence is located _____, _____, California. _____ lived in that home until _____, ____, _____.

3. _____ is currently residing at _____ located at _____, _____, California. However, _____ intends to return home based on my personal knowledge of _____ desire to return home if and when _____ is medically able to return home.

4. Consequently, the principle residence, located at _____, _____, California is, and continues to be an exempt asset. I now have an ownership interest in the residence, and I will maintain the home for _____. _____ will be permitted to return to live at the home whenever _____ wishes and it is medically feasible to do so.

I declare under the penalty of perjury under the laws of the State of California that the foregoing is true and correct and that this Affidavit was executed on the _____ day of _____, _____.

_____
RECIPIENT OF THE PROPERTY

ACKNOWLEDGEMENT

STATE OF CALIFORNIA   )
COUNTY OF _____)

On _____, _____, before me, _____, Notary Public, personally appeared _____, personally known to me-or-proved to me on the basis of satisfactory evidence to be the person(s) whose name(s) is/are subscribed to the within instrument and acknowledged to me that he/she/they executed the same in his/her/their authorized capacity(ies), and that by his/her/their signature(s) on the instrument the person(s), or the entity upon behalf of which the person(s) acted, executed the instrument.

WITNESS my hand and official seal.

_____

PROMISSORY NOTE

_____ DATE $_____

The undersigned promises to pay to the order of _____

the total sum of ($_____) on demand with interest in the amount

of _____ (_____%) on said sum annually until said sum

is paid in full.

                              DATE:_____

                              _____
                                        (signature)

ABOUT THE AUTHORS
F. DOUGLAS LOFTON & MELLANESE S. LOFTON

F. Douglas Lofton is an elder law attorney and stockbroker who practices primarily in the areas of Medi-Cal Planning and Living Trusts. Mr. Lofton is a 1988 graduate from the University of Texas School of Law in Austin, Texas. Mellanese Lofton is an elder law attorney who practices primarily in the areas of Conservatorships and Probate. Mrs. Lofton is a 1974 graduate of the University of California's Boalt Hall, School of Law.

Attorneys F. Douglas Lofton and Mellanese S. Lofton are currently the mother-and-son partners of Lofton & Lofton, a law firm dedicated to providing legal services to the elderly and their caregivers. In addition, F. Douglas Lofton and Mellanese S. Lofton conduct statewide and national educational seminars and in-service training programs for senior citizens, family caregivers, nurses, social workers, lawyers, financial planners, and other professionals and non-professionals who serve the elderly. Lofton & Lofton is located in Benicia, California.

For further information, the Loftons can be reached at: 707.745.1362 or on the Internet: http://www.medi-caladvantage.com or loftons@pacbell.net

N O T E S